THE
PRIMAL BRAIN
SOLUTION

The Evolutionary Approach to Brain Health: Increase Performance, Heal Injury & Avoid Disease

Jennifer Aguilar, MHEd, CBFC

First Printing, 2018

ISBN 978-0692088654

Jennifer Aguilar, MHEd, CBFC
Tucson, AZ 85745
www.jenniferaguilar.net

TABLE OF CONTENTS

NOTE TO READERS

This publication contains the ideas and opinions of its author. It is intended to provide helpful and informative material on the subject of brain health. It is sold with the understanding that the author and publisher are not engaged in rendering medical, health, or any other kind of personal professional services in the book. The reader should consult his or her medical, health, or other competent professional before adopting any of the suggestions in this book or drawing inferences from it.

The author and publisher specifically disclaim all responsibility for any liability, loss, risk, personal or otherwise, which is incurred as a consequence, directly or indirectly, of the use and application of any of the contents of this book.

"If you always put limit on everything you do, physical or anything else. It will spread into your work and into your life. There are no limits. There are only plateaus, and you must not stay there, you must go beyond them."

BRUCE LEE

CHAPTER I

THE BRAIN ON FIRE

You can't see it, feel it or touch it. But this one organ holds the key to your life. Who you are is modulated by the brain, who you could be is controlled by the brain as well. Every other organ, from heart to liver to ovaries, is directly affected by how the brain is functioning. Three pounds of gelatinous, miraculous material and about forty five miles of nerves work night and day to make our extremely complex selves operate. And make no mistake, we are complex.

I never thought too much about my brain. Obviously, it was and is working. But, it seemed like something that's inaccessible. I grew up in a time when people believed the brain was static; once we were done growing nothing new happened. Wow, how wrong that idea was! I grew up, went to college, owned a business, had kids and even by then, I didn't think much about their brains either. I do love my children, and I knew their brain was in there doing its thing (thank goodness!), but it was nothing I had my attention on. I had seen a couple of bad concussions with some friends who played football in high school. They seemed to 'get over it'. We now know this isn't true and those same friends are suffering from the beginning stages of Parkinson's and CTE now. Before I knew what I know now, I dealt with brain fog and forgetfulness the way many of us do - caffeine! All in all, I knew very little about the one organ that drives our existence. This changed dramatically in 2013 when my twelve-year-old suffered his first head injury. He then proceeded to suffer two more head injuries over the next two years. Yes, I agree with you, that is ridiculous! Although he was healthy and the injuries were not 'major', he didn't bounce back like a healthy kid seemingly should. He didn't just 'get over it'. Sadly, the doctors we saw had no answers or solutions. People talked to me about my son's 'new normal' (headaches, light sensitivity, nausea during car rides, limited physical capacity) and although it's years later, I wouldn't recommend saying that to me even now. I wanted his 'old normal'- all of his potential - available to him again. I had one massive, driving question:

Why is my healthy child not recovering from minor head injuries?

It made no sense to me. Healthy people heal from injury, even bad injuries like broken limbs and major surgery. I know of kids that have recovered from leukemia with less symptoms than my son had from hitting his head. There was something wrong, much deeper than his injuries. This book is all about what I discovered.

Your brain is on fire and I don't mean that in a good way. Maybe you know this because you're already struggling, have had an injury (or multiple), or maybe you are afraid of the too-numerous-to-name neurological diseases that are attacking us and people we love. Or perhaps you want to be absolutely the best version of you possible, and you know that starts with the brain. *The Primal Brain Solution* is the antidote to the inflamed modern brain. Make no mistake - your brain is under attack. Mine too. One in ten people have Alzheimer's in the U.S.

That number will go up forty four percent by the year 2025. Someone sustains a brain injury every twelve seconds. Many of those brain-injured people, even those with 'just a concussion', will experience post-concussion syndrome (PCS) where symptoms don't subside or clear up. Neurological disease (migraines, sleep disorders, strokes, MS) costs $800 billion dollars every year and rates of disease are rising in all categories in both the U.S. and Europe. This neurological decline goes hand-in-hand with what Chris Kresser (author of *Unconventional Medicine*) calls a "slow-motion plague" of preventable, chronic disease. One in three people have prediabetes or diabetes. About one in six have autoimmune disease. You probably know about the obesity epidemic, but did you know men's sperm counts have fallen since the 1970s? Did you know that one in forty-five children fall somewhere on the Autism spectrum? And the human brain is actually losing volume and no one knows why. These are often referred to as the diseases of civilization. Modern life, while offering us many benefits, is simply eroding human health. And it is definitely corrosive to brain health. From our exposure to chemicals (and we all have them) to our stressful lifestyles, from overuse of artificial light to our sedentary behavior, we have too many factors working against our human body system and we are paying the price via preventable, degenerative disease. Your brain, and mine, are not immune to this cascade of health disruptors.

If you do nothing, the statistics win. You need a plan, and it starts with brain health. We actually can access this complex organ by understanding how we evolved to be what we are and what our brain is expecting life to be like in order to be robust and healthy.

At the time of my son's first head injury, like most of us, I knew very little. And I knew next to nothing, not just about the brain, but about all the factors that can diminish brain health, so we were at a loss. At first. After his second injury, and subsequent PCS, I dove into the research, I started looking for answers. Why? Because typical medicine, even one of the best concussion clinics for kids, had nothing to offer us that helped. So, I spoke to other parents and veterans and I read about brain anatomy and function. We experimented with different approaches and paid attention to what worked. It took me way too long to start piecing his puzzle together. He suffered for it. I truly do not want one other person to lag behind, to suffer for a year or years because this simple and critical information is too slow to percolate into the culture or even into medicine. This book isn't long. It isn't super technical, but it will give you the basic tools to help heal brain injury, increase mental performance and avoid nasty brain-diseases.

I want you to have the shortcut we didn't have.

So how should your brain feel and operate? What does it look like if something is wrong? If you've just had a head injury, it's probably fairly obvious that something is wrong. If that head injury was seven years ago, you may be missing the connection between your current symptoms and the original brain injury, which is far more common than people think. If you had a chemical exposure twelve years ago and you still don't know about it, there is no way you are looking at brain health as the source of your ills. If you work with computers in an enclosed space for more than six hours a day, you may not be thinking that your inability to sleep well and your daily 3:00 PM energy crash has something to do with diminished brain function. If you are a woman hitting menopause, you may not know that this process changes the brain - this is also true if you just had a baby. If you have or had addiction problems, you probably haven't considered how your brain was affected and what you can do now to heal it. Or you are scared there is nothing you can do.

Almost no one is looking at brain health. This problem is called WNL (We're Not Looking). When your brain is on fire - inflamed and suffering - the symptoms will show up differently in each person. We are all neuro-individuals and the brain is complex, so symptoms can and do range far and wide. And symptoms are truly the best indicator of brain issues that are undetectable via our current diagnostics (MRI and CT) - and most brain problems have no reliable, tech-based diagnostic equipment. It is hard to believe, but there is no diagnostic test for a concussion, there is no blood-test for Alzheimer's or Parkinson's and no one can tell you if you're actually suffering from CTE (chronic traumatic encephalopathy). In fact, MRI and CT are not medically recommended for the vast majority of concussions and brain injuries. We only see the inclusion of imaging for diagnosis when there is serious damage suspected. Exposure to mold that leads to a toxic brain injury (yes, this happens) certainly cannot be diagnosed via any of our modern scanning tools. A CT can see certain things, but not much, and only recently has a diagnostic tool that can be used on live people been discovered for CTE (chronic traumatic encephalopathy). There are also SPECT (single photon emission computed tomography) scans which are used by the famous brain doctor, Dr. Daniel Amen, and there are PET scans. These are helpful to some degree, in some situations. But they fall woefully short of even being able to diagnose why someone suffers from, say, migraines.

Symptoms, self-awareness, paying attention, taking a history, putting the puzzle together is truly the only way to figure this whole brain-thing out. In Appendix One I have a sample of a side-by-side timeline that can help clarify events and symptoms and their relationship. The list below is a wide generalization and not complete by any means, but it can give you a picture of what an unhealthy brain looks and feels like, as well as what parts of the brain are most likely involved with specific symptoms.

Possible Brain Symptoms

General Brain-Dysfunction Symptoms

- Brain-fatigue/energy crashes
- Moodiness/Emotional swings
- Concentrations problems
- ADD/ADHD-like symptoms
- Sleep problems (too much or too little)
- Hormonal dysregulation
- Forgetfulness/memory loss
- Headaches
- Depression and/or anxiety
- Sensitivity to light, movement and/or sound
- Persistent digestive issues
- Ear ringing
- Dizziness or balance issues
- And much, much more

See the lists below for specific symptoms as they are associated to regions of the brain.

Symptoms of Frontal Lobe Damage/Problems

- Loss of physical movement
- Inability to plan
- Loss of spontaneity in interacting with people and/or loss of flexibility in thinking
- Mood changes/instability
- Changes in social behavior (i.e. increased aggression)

Symptoms of Parietal Lobe Damage/Problems

- Loss of writing ability and /or problems with reading
- Difficulty in distinguishing left from right
- Trouble doing mathematics
- Inability to focus visual attention

Symptoms of Occipital Lobe Damage/Problems

- Problems with vision
- Difficulty locating objects
- Trouble identifying colors
- Hallucinations
- Inability to recognize words

Symptoms of Temporal Lobe Damage/Problems

- Difficulty recognizing faces
- Trouble understanding other people's speech

- Short term memory loss
- Increased and/or decreased interest in sexual behavior
- Increased aggressive behavior

Symptoms of Brain-Stem Damage/Problems

- Problems with swallowing
- Difficulty with organization/perception of the environment
- Problems with balance and movement
- Dizziness and nausea

Symptoms of Cerebellum-Area Damage/Problems

- Loss of ability to coordinate movements
- Inability to grab objects
- Tremors and/or dizziness
- Slurred Speech

Keep in mind that diagnosing any issue within the brain is not easy. WNL - We're Not Looking is part of the problem. Rarely is the brain considered during a doctor's visit if the problem is anxiety, depression, weight gain or brain fog. The list of symptoms above is the most reliable tool we have to figure out what is going on in the brain, unless we are looking for a brain tumor or some other structural abnormality, for which MRI and CT are great tools. For the more common brain problems such as insomnia, depression, weight gain, low performance and brain fog there is zero screening and no diagnostic tools. As a culture, we have a host of medications and surgeries to deal with each and every symptom, approaching maladies from an atomistic instead of holistic viewpoint, treating symptoms not causes. Western medicine excels at breaking down organ, cellular and hormonal systems into their tiniest functions and their smallest parts. Unfortunately, after such intense focus, these systems are seen as separate. Consider obesity: In the U.S. about forty percent of adults are considered obese (with a BMI [body mass index] of thirty or higher). There are approximately fifty-nine 'obesity' medications currently on the market and at least twelve different surgeries performed to treat obesity. Yet on the horizon, it looks like the gut biome (bacteria in the gut) is at least partially responsible for how much we weigh. What else affects weight? Social relationships. Virus load. Hormone dysregulation. Artificial light exposure. Toxin exposure. Brain injury. So viewing obesity in this atomistic way as if it were separate from total health, as if life experiences don't affect weight, isn't useful or efficacious. When we look at the brain, we cannot separate it from the rest of our health. We can't blow off insomnia as an isolated issue with 'sleep'. You can take a drug to knock yourself out, but they have multiple side-effects, and will not contributing to overall health. They don't solve the problem in the long run. Like many other organs, the brain has a clock and cleans up at night while we rest, so when we don't sleep, our brain can't complete its cleaning processes. Brain malfunction can cause sleep disruptions, and sleep disruptions caused by external issues like too much screen-time at night can definitely cause brain problems. It's not a one-way system. Nothing is.

When we *do* look, we learn that the diagnoses of brain dysfunction are based on self-reported or observed symptoms (the side-by-side timeline in Appendix One can help with this process). This is the most accurate way to assess each situation. Even the standard, physical neurological test that almost all doctors are trained to deliver in-office an fail on the larger scale. My son passed this test and was cleared as being 'normal' long before his symptoms were gone. The test simply didn't account for the multiple, debilitating experiences he was having everyday! Mild dizziness, headaches, light and sound sensitivity, and depression apparently didn't count. All the information doctors needed in order to clear him was that he could respond to the test, his reflexes worked, he could talk, remember a couple of things, and could stand on one foot. Talk about low standards!

The other issue with brain symptoms is that they may appear months or even years after the initial injury or exposure. In this scenario, no one (not even the patient) is looking at the brain as the possible source of the problem. The link between TBI (traumatic brain injury) and Parkinson's Disease is a perfect example of this and highlights why being proactive about brain health is critical during the entire lifespan. A TBI early in life is connected to a higher incidence of Parkinson's disease, especially if the injury was accompanied by a loss of consciousness. So in between the initial TBI and the onset of Parkinson's, what is missing?

There are probably many symptoms pointing to future issues, symptoms we *can* treat!

"Never let the future disturb you. You will meet it, if you have to, with the same weapons of reason which today arm you against the present."

MARCUS AURELIUS

CHAPTER 2

OUR DIMINISHED BRAINS

I talk a lot about brain injury, but this book is also for people who want better brain performance or to avoid the all-too-common brain diseases that affects us as we get older. So you might be asking, why focus on injury? I use brain injury as a window to see how the brain works and what it needs, what it responds to. There is a lot of research on brain injury. This lens helped me understand what is potentially problematic in our 'normal' brains as well. Neurological issues today are incredibly common and incidence is going up, not down. Research has illuminated a scary little fact: It seems almost all modern people are suffering from some brain diminishment. My son was, and I didn't even know it.

I know you might be saying to yourself, "Come on, everyone's 'brain-injured'? Give me a break!" However, my meta-analysis, which includes a myriad of research from different fields of interest, convinced me that our brains are more susceptible today than ever before. Our brains have diminished in resiliency and are, in fact, shrinking in size (volume). Over the last 10,000 years (which is a blip in history) we've lost about 10% of our brain volume. It's worth noting that I have a particular advantage when it comes to this kind of research - I am not a professional scientist. Yes, in this case it is an advantage! I can look at the information as a whole to include all of the studies, all the anecdotes from any field I want, and draw a holistic picture. Neuroscientists study the function of specific chemicals in the brain, they research brain reactivity or the immune system in the brain (and thank goodness they do!), but they don't hang out with all the other brain scientists all over the world to share their little nook of brain knowledge. They also have to answer to their boss, head of department and research funders - I do not. By accessing their collective results, examining their conclusions I can comb the information to create solutions. So can you. My little book is only a start, I hope many other people get into this and come up with even more efficient and interesting ideas. Let's dive in.

We'll start with brain injury, like I mentioned, because there are 1 million *more* traumatic brain injuries annually than all combined cancer diagnoses (hello!) and more yearly deaths than drug overdose, breast cancer, prostate cancer, or HIV. That's a lot of injury. Someone sustains a brain injury in the U.S. every twelve seconds, and even though participation in organized team sports is *declining*, there are more concussions reported now than in the past. This may be because we have a higher awareness of head injury as a culture, but it may also be that more concussions are happening and that we are having worse symptoms from smaller injuries due to our modern lifestyles that seem directly inhibiting to healthy brain function. On the non-injury side, we know that neurological disorders are increasing, and even though our overall death rate via accident is going down, neurological death rates are rising. It's also important to keep in mind that 'neurological disorders' generally do not include depression, anxiety or panic disorders, even though these are obviously an outcropping of a disordered brain. Brain damage, malfunction and illness is scary. No one wants to talk about it, so we don't. Only recently has there been an increase in awareness with the help of media including the movie *Concussion,* news coverage about NFL players suffering from head injury, and top-level athletes (like snowboarder Kevin Pearce) speaking publicly about his struggles.

This type of injury, illness or imbalance affects the control center of your body and the way you express your mind. Who you are is at risk with even minor damage or changes to the brain. Changes in personality, mood issues and chronic pain all reduce our ability to enact our best selves and to be ourselves in whole. With the knowledge we have now, such as the previously mentioned number of deaths due to brain injury, it's astonishing there isn't more information, better diagnostics and more valid, effective treatments. In fact, it's a medical and cultural oversight of overwhelming proportions.

Children up to age fourteen are the most likely demographic to visit the emergency room for head injury according to the CDC (Centers for Disease Control). The military reported about 28,000 TBIs in 2009 alone. Brain injuries do not heal like other injuries. Recovery is a functional recovery, based on mechanisms that remain uncertain. No two brain injuries are alike and symptoms may appear right away or may not be present for days, weeks, months or years after the injury. Generally speaking, when a brain injury occurs, the brain moves inside the skull causing damage of various forms. Typically in a closed-head injury (when the skull doesn't fracture), damage occurs at the point of contact, although it may also occur on the opposite side of the brain.

Tissue, blood vessels and neural axons can all be torn, bruised or affected. Neural axons link brain cells together and can be described as looking like stringy arms that connect the cells. As I mentioned before, current imaging technology cannot detect all types of brain damage and the point of contact is often not the only area that gets damaged. An open-head injury, such as a gunshot wound where the skull is penetrated, not only creates the same damage as above, but bacteria can be introduced to the brain as well. This is due to whatever force caused the skull to open (i.e. a bullet) leaving the brain literally open to more damage. Patients with open-head injuries have higher mortality rates and are less likely to recover fully, although many do. Every brain injury is totally unique, even in the same person. With the number of ways there are to hit our heads, there are a number of different kinds of injuries. Yet as I mentioned before, blunt force isn't the only injury the brain can sustain.

In addition to sport or accident-sustained brain trauma, chemicals can also cause brain damage and injury. From glues to solvents, lead to pesticides - there are thousands of chemicals that can and do harm the brain. This is often misdiagnosed or missed entirely as people often do not know they were even exposed. The water crisis in Flint, Michigan, where the city switched water sources and inadvertently poisoned the residents with lead, resulted in a fifty-eight percent increase of spontaneous fetal death (death after twenty weeks of pregnancy). Not only were babies dying and no one knew why, women were also incurring brain damage - all from an "invisible" and tasteless source. Chemical causes of brain damage and injury are not only found in big crisis like the one in Flint; they are occurring in what we consider normal, everyday exposures. From new research showing that too much screen time damages the brain (yup) to information on glyphosate (the herbicide chemical in RoundUp) that has been proven to cause negative effects in the brain, we have many points of entry for potential disruptors of proper brain function.

Now that we've covered head and chemical injury, how about what's harming the rest of us? Let's look at this from a specific point of view, from an anthropological and ancestral standpoint. Welcome to the primal part of this book. Our ancient human ancestors sustained concussions and TBIs from falling, combat injuries, violent sports and more, just like we do now. What our ancestors weren't exposed to were vehicle and other high-speed injuries and blast injuries which did not exist for most of human history. So far, we have proven to be a most resilient species (I mean, there are seven billion of us). There is no evidence in the historical record that suggests people in the past recovered better or worse than we do now, but we do know this: The great majority of people in the Western (modern) world are now a sick species and not a healthy, resilient one. Children are suffering from fatty liver disease at ever increasing rates from a diet very high in processed sugars and starches, and older people are suffering from staggering rates of heart disease, diabetes and Alzheimer's. We are not a healthy population, especially in the United States, Britain and Australia (and much of the rest of the world is catching up quickly). This is that slow-motion plague I previously mentioned. If our research about the healthy brain, recovering from head injury or even just basic functioning is based on a population that is sick (and it is), how do we know anything about what is actually possible? How do we know what recovery for a healthy human brain looks like? How do we know what we could feel like? We don't. Or, at least, our information is seriously limited. The situation actually looks even more dire than that, and this is where we come to the problem of diminishment.

Two researchers, Morley and Seneff, proposed in 2014 that many modern people are unknowingly suffering from Diminished Brain Resilience Syndrome (DBRS). The authors explain that DBRS is caused by,

1. Exposure to particular toxins (the authors cite glyphosate and aluminum, among other contaminants)
2. Low nutrition (lack of Omega 3's and critical minerals)
3. Low exposure to sunlight (due to overuse of sunscreen and a more sedentary - indoor - lifestyle)

These issues create a cascade of overreactions in the brain and the brain's immune system, leading to an inability to fully heal from even 'minor' concussions and a host of generalized symptoms in the uninjured population such as sleep issues, brain fog, weight gain and more. When I discovered this information, I had one of many 'a-ha!' moments about my son. This research highlights a population-wide problem, and no one wants to talk about that. This model for understanding how the brain's toxic load and lack of nutrients and sunlight may be causing severe issues in the TBI population is not recognized in mainstream medicine yet, and most practitioners have never heard of DBRS. Certainly, no one has applied it to the general population. It's too scary, too big and what will we do about it anyway? Actually, the authors state (like I do here) that "modifications to lifestyle practices, if widely implemented, could significantly reduce this trend of neurological damage". A little knowledge, some awareness, and a willingness to make changes in behavior can make all the difference to our brain health. I know this to be true, because it is exactly what 'cured' my son.

In case you think your lifestyle is muy perfecto (and kudos to you if you're exercising, spending time outside and trying to eat a healthy diet it does matter!), it's sad to note that we all have exposure to glyphosate (the active ingredient in RoundUp). In research, human urine tests 100% positive for the chemical, while human breast milk tests positive about 30% of the time. Aluminum is also ubiquitous in our lives, found in cookware, vaccines and used as a treatment in our water supply. Sadly for us, these two compounds do not react well in the human brain, causing a host of problems. This is not a political discussion about Monsanto (now owned by and named Bayer Pharmaceuticals), the company that developed and owns RoundUp, it's simply a scientific fact that our brain does not react well when exposed. Period. If we are *all* exposed, we *all* have to do something to negate the effects. This goes for aluminum as well. What about fluoride, which is a known neurotoxin, but used as a dental caries preventative in nearly all city water supplies? Do you know if you've been over-exposed? Have you had your vitamin D levels checked? Do you regularly ingest plenty of DHA (a critical Omega-3 fatty acid)? Almost no one does. As we go through the Primal Protocol, we'll cover all the factors that you can change in order to help increase your body and brain health, reduce toxicity and restore the homeostasis that is normal to humans. I agree completely when Morley and Seneff state, "In its natural state, the body should be able to tolerate disturbances and withstand shocks without collapse, and to recover quickly from injury or illness". This was exactly the answer to my driving question and motivation.

Note: After doing some genetic testing recently for my son, it turns out he has a genetic mutation making him more likely to not be able to process certain chemicals. This may be one reason his head injuries took so much effort to recover from. I look forward to more research in this area.

The reason we are not in that natural state of resilience is most likely directly connected to PDD - Paleo Deficit Disorder. Sounds silly, right? Keep in mind that I don't really think we all have disorders and syndromes, this concept is a quick way to think about a larger problem and serves as a mental shortcut. Rene Dubos, a famed microbiologist, posed long ago that our "progressive loss of contact with natural environments" is affecting our microbiota, immune system and ultimately our lifelong health. Rene stated back in 1970 that "human beings can almost certainly survive and multiply in the polluted cage of technological civilization, but we may sacrifice much of our humanness in adapting to such conditions...The maintenance of biological and mental health requires that technological societies provide in some form the biological freedom enjoyed by our Paleolithic ancestors". Eventually this was called Paleo Deficit Disorder. PDD. You've got it, I have it and our brains suffer for it. A great example from Norman Doidge's book, *The Brain's Way of Healing*, explains that computers and cellphones drive us to use our eyes in a near constant 'central fixation', meaning we're ignoring peripheral activity. Because these devices don't take our biology into account, they cause physical problems and more. Did you know the eyes literally mold our brain and guide its development? Researchers have tracked a protein called Otx2 that travels from the eye to the brain. This protein tells the brain when to become 'plastic' or when to learn. How important do you think that is? Imagine what the overuse of screen time in infants and toddlers is doing to their very plastic brains? Actually, you don't need to imagine because research shows that too much screen time for infants results in speech and hearing delays among other serious problems. What about screen time for adults? Well, WNL, are we?

Let's look at how we've set up our work environments. They don't take into account that we need a lot of movement and sunshine. Sitting is a risk in multiple health factors; usually we are sitting for long periods inside, lacking critical sunlight. Then we might spend our evenings looking at more screens, moving even less and still inside away from the sun. Additionally, we're exposed to indoor air, which typically contains more chemicals and pollutants than outdoor air. Another modern stressor? Much of the disease we see in our population is caused by systemic inflammation from a high-sugar, high-chemical and high-stress lifestyle. These are somewhat controllable factors. Inflammation, like TBI, is the body's response to immediate injury and the overload of certain stressors. Though if inflammation persists, symptoms persist and healing slows or stops completely. Some of the research I've included in this guide points to the benefit of inflammation-reducing supplements, compounds and plants for healing the brain.

While it is really tricky to understand all of the critical functions that happen in the brain (even I don't get it all), there is another issue that precedes inflammation, which is immunoexcitotoxicity. Now, that's a fun word! If you think that sounds bad, it is. When your brain gets overloaded with things that aren't supposed to be there such as glyphosate, too much sugar, alcohol, too many cannabinoids, estrogenic compounds, etc., it considers these things toxic. Add a small brain injury to already present inflammation, and the brain's own immune system goes into overdrive. When this immune system is constantly on alert and working, the brain gets over-excited and this causes serious problems and symptoms. These can include headaches, tremors, and learning disabilities - the symptoms are endless. Morley and Seneff explain it this way, "The interaction between immune receptors within the central nervous system (CNS) and excitatory glutamate receptors triggers a series of events, such as extensive reactive oxygen species/ reactive nitrogen species generation, accumulation of lipid peroxidation products, and prostaglandin activation, which then leads to dendritic retraction, synaptic injury, damage to microtubules, and mitochondrial suppression". Whew! In other words (words you and I can grasp!), the brain cannot fully heal when the brain's immune system is overheating. As you might imagine, the density and complexity of the science of the brain is why I am not going to turn this book into a treatise on brain malfunction. Let's just say that Diminished Brain Resilience Syndrome (DBRS) is a real problem, as is PDD. The good news is that they are (possibly, even mostly) fixable problems.

Finally we come to the gut-brain axis. This is the concept that the gut and brain are deeply connected, affecting each other constantly.

When the brain is injured, the gut bacteria react. Pretty smart, right? Intestinal immune cells travel from the gut to the injured areas of the brain to help with anti-inflammatory efforts. Brilliant! This is where lifestyle and nutrition matter, a lot. Our constant use of antibiotics, lack of good bacteria in the food supply and exposure to chlorine and fluoride all change our body's natural ecosystem in ways we don't fully understand at this juncture. Essentially, it's a reduction of our good load of bacteria and this affects the brain because it can't receive proper support from the body when our gut is not healthy.

This is a modern problem, just like our problem with diabetes, cancer and heart disease. We are less likely to recover well from TBI because we are, as modern, Westernized humans, generally unhealthy. Even without an injury, our brain is under tremendous pressure and exposed to many factors that have never before existed in our species. We are frogs in hot water. Our health has deteriorated over time in so many ways that we just don't notice. We think being ill is normal. We think being obese is normal. We think being constantly medicated is normal, but it's not. If we are susceptible to obesity, high blood pressure, cancer and diabetes, those susceptibilities absolutely leave the brain at risk. It's not a separate organ from the rest of the body. If our modern diet is extremely high in sugar, how is this affecting the brain? How is our exposure to multiple chemicals in the food supply affecting our abilities to heal from TBI? What about our exposure to nnEMFs (non-native electromagnetic frequencies) - WIFI - and RFs (radio frequencies) - cell phones? What about our very low intake of omega-3 fatty acids, which are essential for brain function? You cannot create a healing paradigm within a population that does not even have base-levels of health. And many do not.

What if our ancestors - and I don't mean from the Dark Ages, I mean from 60,000 years ago - fared better than we do with brain injuries because their baseline health was better? What if they didn't suffer from chronic brain disease, or afternoon brain fog or ADHD? A recent study examined the bones of women from 7,000 years ago and found that these women were stronger than elite female athletes of today! They showed no signs of bone loss or osteoporosis and stronger bones mean less bone breaks as well. What other health markers were better in the past? We know that diabetes is a mostly modern disease, and we suspect that cancer is (mostly) as well. Is a lack of physical activity or low vitamin D leading to thinner skulls? Does prediabetes leave the brain more at risk? It makes sense. Most people have no idea they are pre-diabetic, but about eighty-four million adult Americans are. That is why the ancestral viewpoint is so critical. It allows us to change our mind about what we are, change our health and get back our robust human brain by using a primal mindset.

"Delay not, swift the flight of
fortune's greatest favors."

SENECA

CHAPTER 3

WHAT IS THE BRAIN?

Your brain is weird. Mine too. It's also adaptable, powerful and mysterious. Don't worry, this is perfectly normal for us *Homo sapiens*. Brain-organs - and the brain is an organ like the lungs or heart - are strange and unique. Our brain is big (really big!) compared to other animals and it transmits chemical and electrical signals. However, it's mushy and delicate, encased in our bony skull to protect it from harm. The brain has another barrier as well, a membrane that keeps the good stuff in and the bad stuff out. It also has an immune system that is separate from the rest of the body. We have strange mirror neurons that light up when we see others doing certain activities, as if we are doing the activity ourselves. We learn through copying others and this process is also how we empathize (a critical human behavior). What's more, the brain isn't just a dull gray color! Parts of it are black, some are white, and some are pink or red. Imagine a bowl of multi-colored Jello that is electrically charged, can drive a car, attend college and learn Mandarin Chinese. That's essentially us - a miraculous bowl of Jello. The brain is about three pounds of gelatinous, fat-based material that allows us to do everything we do and to be who we are. From our personality to our heartbeat, the brain runs it all. Our brain is a rare organ that allows us to enact our potential as human beings.

When this is endangered by traumatic brain injury, it's terrifying. When our innate capacity is threatened by a brain-toxic landscape that is virtually invisible, it has the potential to change our present moment and our future in severe and harmful ways. This is why it's critical to know what a brain is, and what it isn't, what it needs and what it doesn't. What is done to our brain and what we do with our brain determines everything. Everything. This book is for anyone who wants to brain-hack their way to high performance, to heal brain injury and/or to avoid future brain disease. That's everyone. And the good news is that you do not need to be a neurologist to take care of your brain! You don't need to understand all the complicated - and trust me, it's complicated - processes and structures of the brain.

So why the *Primal Brain*? What is 'primal' anyway? Is it innate, paleo, evolutionary, inherent, functional, ancestral (meaning older than your Grandma), and dare I say 'natural'? Yes, all that and more. The brain is a very old organ. Did you know the first creatures on Earth didn't even have brains? Over millions of years of evolution, the brain emerged and (as it exists today) requires certain things. Our modern lifestyles are leaving each of our brains vulnerable. This book is about how to heal from a brain injury, avoid brain disease and increase brain function (now!) and much, much more. By viewing health and living through an ancestral lens, we can align ourselves with what we are already:

Homo sapiens

Homo sapiens are built to move, create, be social and solve problems. And these capacities and needs were created over a long span of evolution and thousands upon thousands of years of specific experiences like hunting, raising children, migrating, building communities, knowing the foodscape, understanding weather and the movement of the stars, so on and so forth. We could easily be called *Homo socialis* (collaboration is our superpower) or *Homo faber* (creativity is another superpower). Though if we truly want to be wise (*sapien*), then we need to acknowledge where we come from, what we were built for and how we function.

"For more than half a century now, psychologists, linguists, neuroscientists and other experts on human behaviour have been asserting that the human brain works like a computer," Dr. Robert Epstein stated in an essay on the blog, *Aeon*. In his essay, *The Empty Brain*, Dr. Epstein reminds us that we are born with senses, reflexes and learning mechanisms. What we aren't born with is "information, data, rules, software, knowledge, lexicons, representations, algorithms, programs, models, memories, images, processors, subroutines, encoders, decoders, symbols, or buffers". In other words, we are not computers, which is an essential concept in *The Primal Brain Solution*. George Zarkadakis explains in his book, *In Our Own Image*, that we have employed many metaphors for the brain over time, the computer being the most recent. The Greeks thought the brain worked like an aqueduct and that the 'humors' (bile, phlegm and blood) had to be kept in balance. The famous philosopher, Rene Descartes, supposed in the 1600s that the nervous system transported animal spirits to and from the brain. In the middle 1700's, when mechanics were being more widely used in industry, biologists saw the cells as small factories and were taken with a mechanical idea of the brain (gears and levers). When the telegraph and telephone were introduced, the brain was compared to telephone networks and then finally, in our age, to computer processors. So why do we need a metaphor? Because we don't know what it *is* exactly. Weirdly, we have a hard time using our big brain to figure out what our brain actually is.

I bring this up because the very idea - brain = computer - is so ingrained in our current culture, it grossly limits our ability to imagine different solutions for capacity and healing. It also limits what we think our brain needs and our understanding of how it can be harmed. A metaphor that is wrong (or an inaccurate comparison) can close off avenues of inquiry. And it has. It can make us blind to the obvious or limit our imaginings, leaving us without solutions to common problems like concussion- the very, very common problem we don't have a solution for. Isn't it strange, with all of our tech, with all of our knowledge, there is no cure for concussion, parkinson's, Alzheimer's, CTE, ADHD, OCD, anxiety and on and on. *The Primal Brain Solution* is a small step towards changing our metaphor, and therefore our understanding, in order to create a healthier brain for everyone. To hopefully, find cures. Nature is actually where we can find better comparisons to the human brain. Fungi (i.e. mushrooms) have unique and intriguing aspects. Mushrooms grow these masses of tendrils, or thin threads called mycelium. The mycelia connect the fungi underground, but they also connect to the roots of other plants. With these connections they pass around nutrients and information. They can actually sabotage unwanted plants by spreading toxic chemicals through the network. If that's not smart and brainy, I don't know what is! Start thinking of your brain as a big mushroom and you will be closer to reality than thinking about it like it's a computer.

Many of us think that one area of the brain controls one area of our functioning. It's nice and mechanical - straightforward. It's somewhat true, but like most things brain-related, it's more complicated and nuanced than that. Even simple tasks involve multiple regions of the brain and traumatic, difficult or challenging experiences can excite nearly the entire organ. Let us begin to imagine the brain differently. Back in the 1920s a neuroscientist by the name of Karl Lashley determined that facts, skills and other things we 'know' are not stored in individual neurons or in the connections between them. Instead, they exist in what he called "cumulative electrical wave patterns". This is the idea that all of the neurons involved in a specific activity are firing together and wiring together, creating pathways in the brain. If you're a rock climber, every time you chalk up, touch a rock face and start moving your body, the thousands (10s or 100s of thousands - we don't know) of neurons involved in that activity start firing together so you can climb. By continued repetition of the activity, the rock climber creates stronger and stronger neural pathways, recruiting more neurons to carry out the activity which creates an even stronger electrical pattern that is recognized as 'rock climbing'. This phenomenon is known as neuroplasticity. Later, when the rock climber sits down to watch a movie, 'rock climbing' is not activated in the brain because 'rock climbing' is not a solid, physical structure that exists in the brain. Enacting the skill depends on a solid physical structure (neurons, axons, synapses, etc.), but the act itself is an electrical reality. This is why the brain heals the way it does, which is amazing. It's why the brain is so flexible. It's why if you lose the capacity to read because of a head injury, you can probably learn to read again by asking the brain to recruit new/different neuronal networks to carry out the activity, sometimes even from the opposite, undamaged hemisphere.

So it's worth repeating that the brain is not a machine, it is part of an organism - us. It's an amazing biological organ. Columbia University neuroscientist, Erik Kandel, said it will take 100 years to actually understand the human brain! So don't feel stress if it seems hard to grasp - it is. The complicated nature of the brain is why I started from the other end of beast. I started with this idea: What makes a brain healthy and robust? We already know that, it's easy to observe. Much easier than figuring out every aspect of the brain and all its' functions.

The various regions of the brain do have individual jobs, like controlling spatial awareness, but they all work in concert with the other regions, which allows the brain to pretty much use any neuron for any job (and it has 100 billion neurons to play with). Additionally, each person is a neuro-individual, meaning each and every brain operates in its own unique way. This can help explain why each person who has the same physical experience (like a car crash) will report it in completely different ways; or how people learn in varied ways as well through listening, seeing or touching.

Another concept that needs to change is this thinking that the brain is somehow separate from the rest of our body. We assume our brain runs everything and sends out orders like a dictator when in fact, the brain is influenced (a lot!) by all the stimuli we receive as well. From Dr. Doidge's paradigm-shifting book, *The Brain's Way of Healing*, we learn that "a brain cannot think without motor function". Wait, what? To put it simply, we don't have a fully optimized brain without physical movement. In general, evolutionary terms, the brain evolved after the body and it exists to serve the body (you know, so we can physically survive and stuff). Without movement, some parts of the brain fall into non-use. The brain can even shrink and slowly lose function! It takes in impulses from the body, meaning it's not a one-way system. It's not a even a two-way system. We are sensitive to light, electro-magnetics, social interactions and the air we breathe. We are constantly responding to our environment and our own internal cues, simultaneously, all the time.

Furthermore, the brain in our head isn't our only brain. WHAT?! Our heart has its own neural network, and our gut has a very large neural network (the enteric nervous system) composed of approximately 500 million neurons. This is a point worth reading again - our gut contains 500 million neurons, those things that most people assume only live in the brain. This system starts in our esophagus and extends all the way to the anus. In fact, most of the serotonin in our body is produced in the gut, not the brain. Our gut-brain usually talks to our head-brain via the vagus nerve, but will continue to function on its own if it's cut off. Remember when I said the brain is weird? So weird.

The human brain is more complicated than the brains of other mammals and even other primates. We are a sophisticated species with one communicating body system, not separate systems. Our brains evolved over millions of years to operate in a particular way, to remain healthy and adaptable *only* under certain circumstances and to withstand and recover from injury. It evolved to thrive when it's dark at night and light during the day. It evolved to be at its best when the body is in motion. It grew to expect responsiveness and care from other humans. This is the evolutionary view of the brain. Our brain is primal, old, unique, and *The Primal Brain Solution* fits and respects what the brain actually is and how it functions.

"You cannot escape the responsibility of tomorrow by evading it today."

ABRAHAM LINCOLN

CHAPTER 4

IT'S IN OUR HANDS

So why do I even care about the brain? What got me interested? I've always been interested in health. My mom was a master herbalist (she passed away in March 2017). I learned how to meditate when I was five years old, started doing yoga at age ten, and took courses in ayurveda and aromatherapy as a young adult. Before I finished college, I became a childbirth educator and lactation counselor. After my first two (of four) children were born, I returned to college and earned my BA (in human development) with a concentration in pre and perinatal psychology and health. I finished my MS in health education after my fourth child was born, and afterwards became a community health and parent educator. I then furthered my education by taking the intensive Parents as Teachers (PAT) certification. At home, I experimented with diet and lifestyle, always refining my knowledge through reading, listening to podcasts and watching documentaries. Even now, I am always engaged in studying something - I love learning (hint, this habit is great for the brain)!

My intensive focus on brain health, however, began when my 14 year-old son lay on a gurney in the emergency room, contusions on his face, shoulder separated and brain bleeding after crashing his bike in a skate park. Yes, he had a helmet on - people always ask. That was the catalyst, and while it was hellish, it also led to this book. It was my son's third (that's right!) traumatic brain injury in two years, which is an alarming number of injuries to the brain in that amount of time. The doctors in our rural mountain town were concerned enough to put us on an emergency flight to a larger hospital with a pediatric intensive-care unit (ICU) and neurologist. His second TBI, about a year earlier, caused nearly a year of post-concussion syndrome (PCS) where debilitating symptoms continued long after the injury. I knew he could not tolerate another year of suffering and in that bright, loud emergency room I made a commitment to make sure he wouldn't suffer like that again. My protocol for the brain is a product of the accidental journey we took. My personal experience, that includes extensive research and my work as a consultant with numerous clients healing brain injury/disease and increasing brain performance, led to this protocol. About two weeks after my son's third accident, while following my customized protocol for healing the brain, my son was back in the rock climbing gym, going low and slow. At three weeks post-trauma, he was able to attend a bouldering competition- not as a true competitor; his goal was to attend, not to win. Under two weeks later he was reading books again, and then finally, after twelve months, he could run again with zero symptoms. He suffered no depression, very few headaches, only mild concentration issues, very few angry outbursts, no ringing in the ears, no visual problems, and only very mild aphasia. All in all, he has recovered from all three TBIs. We still work on some small symptomatology that pops up now and then under pressure but are able to address these issues with confidence. We believed he could heal, were aggressive in his treatment and followed an 'alternative path' that isn't actually alternative at all- it's evolutionary, ancestral. The protocol in this book is a cohesive and comprehensive version of the experimental approach we adopted for my son's healing. My knowledge about how to heal TBI, concussion, and PCS comes first-hand through my own experiences and extensive meta-analysis where I examined and interpreted as much research on the brain as I could. My experimentation and study led to my learning about how to increase my own brain performance as well. Although I was already a health coach and writer, it's my role as a parent that motivated me to learn why my son was so susceptible to the lingering effects of brain injury and how to help him heal his brain.

You might assume that the brain is too complicated to effectively learn how to heal it without being a neurologist, but I found this isn't the case. There is so much you can do at home, on your own, or by working with specific practitioners to get more functionality from your brain. To heal, completely by understanding what the brain needs to be healthy. This is possible and the information is accessible because what I present here is all based on evolutionary and ancestral biology. Today we live with many evolutionary mismatches; our modern lifestyle doesn't match what we have evolved to do, be or to eat. An evolutionary mismatch is essentially where your biology, and what it needs, runs into something that doesn't match that need. For example, many of us sit for most of the day working on computer screens. This behavior doesn't match what we evolved to do (move, run, jump, walk) and we suffer for it. My approach is really just a commonsensical approach. I began by assuming that as your body wants to heal a cut (and it does), the brain wants to heal and has ways to do that. According to the research and data I studied, this turns out to be true. I also assumed that I would be able to figure it out by first becoming a student in various fields of research, and then closely following the rules of nature. We are biological creatures living on this planet, and our optimal functioning happens within the physical laws of Earth. Unfortunately it's just too easy for modern, industrialized people to forget that simple fact. Consider this note written by Florence Nightingale,

> *"It is the unqualified result of all my experience with the sick, that second only to their need of light; after a closed room, what hurts them most is a dark room, and it is not only light but direct sunlight that they want....People think that the effect is upon the spirit only. This is by no means the case. The sun is not only a painter but a sculptor." -*
> *Notes on Nursing, 1860*

The famous nurse wrote this after observing that men in her care healed faster if she made sure they got to sit in the sun each day. She may not have known about Vitamin D, but nature did. It plays a critical role in many healing processes, and is highly beneficial to the brain. Unfortunately, the current Western medical narrative about the human brain is limited. It certainly doesn't include considering sunlight's effects on brain healing, or how much screen-time might be affecting sleep and mood. Most neurologists don't ask patients about their intake of sugar or DHA (an essential fatty acid), and most often it's because medical institutions themselves don't require our doctors and neurologists to learn about the effects of nutrition on healing. That's just one avenue we need to explore further.

The Human Brain Project (started in 2013) is an international effort by scientists to use all the information we have globally to create a working model of the brain. Living in a technologically advanced culture, it's easy to believe we know a lot about the brain and how it heals, but we don't. Research is ongoing and our understanding of how the brain works and heals is increasing, but certainly not complete. In his essay, *Neuralink and the Brain's Magical Future*, blogger Tim Urban starts off with a truth that, "This ridiculous-looking thing [the brain] is the most complex known object in the universe—three pounds of what neuro-engineer Tim Hanson calls 'one of the most information-dense, structured, and self-structuring matter known,' all while operating on only 20 watts of power [an equivalently powerful computer runs on 24,000,000 watts]".

One example that highlights our low-level understanding of the brain is the fact that researchers are just now learning about the intimate connection between our gut bacteria and our brain, which I previously discussed. This critical feature of our human function was completely unseen and unknown until quite recently. Researchers now know that Parkinson's Disease actually starts in the gut, and there is new evidence that ADHD may be a type of sleep disorder. Imagine what else we don't know! As good research continues to give us better models of biological functioning to work from, we can be thankful. However, we need to keep in mind that right now it is likely we do not understand or even know of something that will one day be proven critical to our health! Something equivalent to the concept of our gut biome is hiding within us, waiting for our discovery. That's why understanding what your biology needs to be healthy in the first place is important. It's also simple and will move faster than research will. It's a holistic understanding of your entire system. You don't need to be a specialist in mitochondrial function to get better brain performance, to heal a brain injury, to have more energy, or to lose weight.

Why? It's the power of the non-expert. It's the power of evolution. We don't need more data or research to know how to heal the human body. Trusting what's been passed down over thousands of years, aligning with your biology and with how you evolved - with what you are already - is enough for most problems. Not all, but most. Our amazing tech, our cutting-edge meds can be reserved for our toughest cases; situations where a person wouldn't have recovered or survived in the past. For the rest of us, addressing our daily evolutionary mismatches is enough to swing us into a virtuous cycle of health. And it's not that hard.

Initially, people with TBI may need surgery, blood transfusions, fMRI, CT, PET or other diagnostics, physical therapy, pharmaceuticals for seizures and pain medication. Each and every incident that leads to brain injury is markedly different. From an IED explosion to a collision on the soccer field to chemical exposure - the initial treatments can vary widely. If symptoms don't abate within a reasonable period of time, patients are usually encouraged to take anti-depressants, anti-seizure drugs, steroid injections and other pharmaceuticals in addition to cognitive behavior therapy and physical therapy. Here is where we come (essentially) to the end of standard western medical treatment. This is a problem because diet/nutrition, supplements, herbs, light therapy and lifestyle changes and other 'alternative' (remember, they are ancestral, not alternative) treatments are valid, helpful treatments for healing the brain (and body!). See the reference section, which is loaded with relevant science regarding these supposed alternatives. That is not to say western medicine, especially emergency medicine, does not have a place and is not valuable. It certainly is! Though as David Epstein wrote in his excellent article, *When Evidence Says No, But Doctors Say Yes*, "It is distressingly ordinary for patients to get treatments that research has shown are ineffective or even dangerous".

Mr. Epstein goes on to give one of the best examples of how the application of medicine doesn't often follow current research, or even common sense, and is operating from a mechanical point of view which misses critical pieces about how the brain operates and heals. His example goes as follows: Deep brain stimulation (DBS, in which electrodes are placed inside the brain) is sometimes used to alleviate symptoms in people who are suffering from Parkinson's disease (PD). The first study conducted showed that DBS improved spatial memory in PD patients, but the study size was small, just seven people. Researchers attempted to replicate the findings in a larger group of forty-nine people. Their findings? DBS actually impairs spatial memory, but it can improve the tremors of PD. Unfortunately, the risks from DBS are as high as the risk of brain surgery (because essentially it is brain surgery). There is also a twenty percent hardware failure rate in DBS treatments leading to prolonged antibiotics, hospitalization and repeat surgery. The first study was published in the New England Journal of Medicine and the second study was rejected *by the same journal*, which is important for us to be aware of because it means the second study's more legitimate findings never made it to mainstream medical professionals. And I already mentioned that Parkinson's seems to start with gut dysbiosis, so direct mechanical treatments are probably unnecessary and will be seen (in the future) as barbaric.

All doctors are not created equally. You may be seeing a doctor that stays educated using current research, but her hands are clinically tied as a result of her hospital not investing in newer equipment. Or maybe, your doctor does not keep up with current research. Maybe he keeps up, but keeps doing the same surgeries because they are lucrative. There are as many scenarios as there are doctors. The problem here isn't your individual doctor, but that our culture's conception of the brain isn't accurate. We depend on drugs and surgery when other pathways are proven to work better. We see this in research on healing brain injury through light, sound, nutrition and physical therapies. The same actually applies to most of our common, but not normal, modern diseases. We apply drugs and surgery to many diseases (and many non-diseases) that respond well to lifestyle and nutritional intervention. It's a mistake of gargantuan proportions with financial, societal and community fallout.

Another troubling fact is that western doctors and practitioners are not clinically trained or educated in natural, healthy lifestyle habits. They do not study nutrition in depth, how sunlight affects brain health (and it does), how artificial light disrupts circadian rhythms (this has powerful negative effects) and most have very little training in the relationship between dietary fat intake and brain health. If you can't sleep, there are pills for that. If you have low vitamin D, you simply take more, with zero acknowledgement that the brain and the eyes have photoreceptors and need actual sunlight (when available).

If you want to heal, if you want to reach your potential, then you have to move beyond the western paradigm which is a surgery and drug-based system that falls woefully short for most people with brain injury, diminishment and disease. Our current system utterly fails to address those who want better brain function or to achieve higher performance. In fact, we could argue that most people don't realize this is even an option. Hippocrates was correct in observing that "natural forces within us are the true healers of disease," and this book was born from the simple fact that we are self-healing organisms. When your brain isn't operating at it's best, when you need more focus and power in order to grow (a new business or a new skill), for kids who need to do better in school and succeed in the real world, when the TBI patient returns home and doctors have exhausted their initial efforts, when PCS stretches on and on and allopathic medicine has done what it can do - The Primal Protocol has answers. Ultimately, it's in our hands and there are solutions! We will harness these solutions using our primal functions and our obligate needs to help the body restore the brain to balance.

"Part of the healing process is
sharing it with other people
who care."

JERRY CANTRELL

CHAPTER 5

HOW THE BRAIN HEALS

The brain has a remarkable capacity to heal itself. We call this neuroplasticity. B. Bethune states in *How Your Brain Heals Itself*, "The brain is actually a supple, malleable organ, as ready to unlearn as it is to learn, capable of transforming vicious circles into virtuous circles, of resetting and repairing its internal communications". Whether we understand the processes or not, it's easy to observe. This is the foundation upon which this book is written. The inherent, built-in nature of the brain to heal is what we are relying on here. In Dr. Norman Doidge's book, *The Brain's Way of Healing*, he says, "We see patients in whom years of chronic pain have been alleviated, and others who have recovered the ability not just to walk or talk but to live fully despite debilitating strokes, as well as cases of long-standing brain injuries cured or vastly improved.". JJ Virgin's book, *The Miracle Mindset*, is about her son's recovery from life-threatening TBI (among other serious injuries caused by a hit-and-run accident). In the end, it's really about having the mindset to heal, to allow for what we think is a miracle to happen. The funny thing is that the brain seems to be really, really good at miracles. Maybe what we think is amazing is just par for the course in Brain Land?

Considering that not long ago we viewed the brain as a non-changeable, rigid organ, this notion isn't too far-fetched. Over and over again we've seen hypotheses in science that we think are 'settled' crumble as new minds pose better questions or develop superior techniques (thank you, scientific method!). Whatever we think we know now, will eventually evolve, change or be disproven. What is powerful about the *Primal Brain Solution* is that it is not dependent on new science. In some ways, knowing the science isn't important to heal your brain, like I said before. If you want to be become a brain-nerd, go for it! There is a huge body of research and plenty of room for up and coming neurologists and neuroscientists. But, just knowing that it *can* heal and *how* to push it into a virtuous cycle is truly all that is critical. Before we discuss how the brain heals, I would ask that you develop a mental shield to protect yourself from beliefs that are mistaken about the brain. No matter who the person is (doctor, friend, scientist) that tells you healing is limited, or that two years after a TBI nothing new can happen or that whatever disability is permanent, or that you cannot prevent neurological diseases or heal them - build a stone wall and never let those beliefs in!

They are so often wrong.

Here are the basic brain-healing components:

Healing/Performance Premise #1
Use It or Lose It

That is a literal statement! The less activity you engage in - both physically and mentally - the less volume your brain will have and the looser the connections. What you want is a heavy brain with tight neural connections - thick, dense, heavy, robust. The brain absolutely depends on behavior, activity, environment and movement to regain lost capacity or to change a vicious cycle (say, headaches) into a virtuous cycle (no headaches). Rehabilitative therapy (RT) is one avenue people pursue to engage in the process of brain remodelling. It's critical to enlist the brain in everything you want it to do. No matter what that function is, this is how you get it back, improve it or learn something utterly new. The process of doing this is based on the neuro-individuality of each person. Everyone learns differently, at different rates and has various issues to overcome. Plasticity is learning and learning is uncomfortable. Get comfortable with discomfort and your learning rate will skyrocket, as will your ability to problem-solve your own brain problems.

Healing/Performance Premise #2
The Brain Needs Critical Nutrients

We are biological organisms, and that means our cells (our bodies) require specific elements to survive. The brain has specific needs that must be met (especially if it is working to heal itself). This is a short list of common nutrients we know are low in most modern people. There are no nutrients that are not critical to the brain! But, here is a short-list of neuro-critical nutrients:

- Magnesium
- Omega-3 Fatty Acids
- Vitamin D
- Vitamin E

- Vitamin C
- All the B vitamins - B6, B12, Thiamine, Riboflavin (B2), Niacin, Folate
- Saturated Fats
- Probiotics
- Quality Proteins
- Iron
- Copper
- Zinc

Healing Premise #3
Lifestyle Matters

Lifestyle is a make it or break it issue for a healthy brain. Things like stress-load, sunlight exposure, physical movement, relationship interactions, amount and quality of sleep, type of work or schooling, total daily screen time and environmental toxin exposure can all have positive or negative effects on the human brain. If you want to tip your brain into a virtuous cycle (get it to heal, perform better, be less anxious, etc.) these issues must be addressed.

Healing Premise #4
You Are the Director of Your Neuroplasticity

You can and must use your own mind to heal your own brain. Funny, right? Active awareness of vicious patterns and conscious attempts to change those patterns does work to heal the brain. It's amazing! It's also hard work. And, for those who are severely compromised, another human being needs to be the director of your neuroplasticity. That's why great care providers, people who push you, physical therapists, psychological therapists, functional medicine doctors and others can help create a great team that in turn, gets the healing cycle going.

"You must be passionate, you
must dedicate yourself, and you
must be relentless in the pursuit of
your goals. If you do, you will
be successful."

STEVE GARVEY

CHAPTER 6

CHANGING THE PARADIGM & BEING RELENTLESS

My viewpoint is clear: I assume that a healthy person can completely heal from TBI, concussion, OCD, anxiety, headaches, brain fog, palsy and even early Parkinson's and Alzheimer's. Can everyone recover? No. But I believe you can cure brain fog and reverse some brain degenerative diseases (caught early enough). I believe that we can recapture lost brain health and vibrance. I believe we are supposed to be intelligent, have clarity, feel good, experience positive emotions and that low-level, persistent symptoms are not normal - even if they are common. This is critical to my approach. When doctors told me that my son's healing (from his third TBI) would take six months to two years, I was not really listening because I knew we didn't (and still don't) live a 'typical' American life and thus do not have many of the poor health markers found in our society. I knew how to enact the lifestyle, diet and neuroplastic training to help him heal. Plus, I am just incredibly stubborn when it comes to my kids.

Rates of disease and prescription drug use continue to rise in our country. The number of children on multiple prescription drugs continues to increase along with the obesity and childhood disease epidemics (i.e. diabetes and myopia). Our 'healthcare' system is a sick-care system, and as a health educator I know one thing: If you want to be healthy and free of disease, you better take control of your health, because our system is not there to optimize your health. This process starts with what you believe. It's not esoteric, it's that most people have truly limited beliefs about what is possible and a low understanding of their own biology. Including not understanding the power of neuroplasticity and their own power within that system. We might not even know what it feels like to be fully in our own capacity- to be really healthy.

People with brain symptoms or injury are surrounded by a culture that believes healing is not possible or necessary. The only solution is drugs or accepting a lifetime of headaches and angry outbursts. Our culture tries to manage the symptoms, not heal or fix the problems. In that paradigm, how is total healing possible? How is potential reachable? It's not. Your own mind is your most powerful tool for healing. In *The Brain's Way of Healing*, Dr. Doidge (obviously, I'm a big fan) explains that instead of seeing the patient as "a helpless bystander," like many doctors do, the neuroplastician "require[s] the active involvement of the whole patient in his or her own care: mind, brain, and body." Do I think you can just think or pray your way to a healed brain? No, physical action is necessary - your effort is required. We are physical beings after all. Yet without the right mindset, physical efforts are not enough. In fact, we are looking to use the body and mind to *treat* the brain. Brilliant, no? The brain is not separate or above the body and mind. Remember, the brain evolved after bodies did (initially) - to serve the body! I mentioned earlier that gut health affects brain functioning, and that is because the brain is listening to all of the body and responding to it. The brain-body connection is a two-way relationship with the mind (the element of you that is conscious, experiences the world and gives you a sense of self) being the imperial ruler over all. If the mind is employed to heal the brain, amazing things can happen.

As I mentioned before, my son, was a few days from his fourteenth birthday when he had his third head injury within two years. The first one was a concussion caused by wrestling with Dad in the living room. The second, three months later, was a bike accident in front of the house, with his helmet on. It took seven months to recover from that one, with fairly severe post-concussion syndrome (PCS). We tried everything to attempt to lift him out of the fog, and nothing worked until my learning caught up to his problems and we implemented a beta-test of the Primal Protocol. For the third injury, he was riding his bike at the skatepark, braked too hard on an incline and went over the bike, landing on his face. He had a separated shoulder, facial and mouth contusions, lacerations, and intraparenchymal hemorrhage (a small bleed in the brain, leading to the diagnosis of TBI). We called 911 and the ambulance took him to the local emergency room where a CT and x-rays were conducted to assist with diagnoses. Here is where we digress from the 'standard'.

Because he lost consciousness at the scene and had difficulty coming around, I knew his head was affected well before the diagnoses. I also knew his concussion history (the doctors did not), and I knew he was adverse to needles and hospitals (leftover psychological issues from the other injuries). I knew he had great fear and paranoia of having another head injury and suffering through PCS again. Wouldn't you? It sucks! The months of PCS were absolute torture for him. While he was passed out on the table in the emergency room, I started talking to him. I repeated these things, out loud, over and over again:

- You will heal 100% from this injury
- You will heal very quickly
- Your body is already healing

Why did I do this? Because I believed that he was still 'present' and available to receive these messages. He needed a strong mind to lean on. His brain was working, just mildly injured. I knew now that his mind would be master over his injuries and there was no way in hell I was going to allow him to fall back into PCS or not recover 100% from this injury. Did I mention I am stubborn when it comes to my kids? This was not an option. This is mindset work, it's employing the mind to heal the brain and body. Mindset is everything. If you don't know why your brain is foggy, or you're depressed, or have headaches - this is where you start.

For myself, I was also using mindset work. If I allowed myself to collapse into despair, how would I be of help to him? How would I be creative in problem-solving his injury? How would parent my other children with positivity? The discipline of maintaining a growth and positive mindset is hard. It takes work. And, yes, every once in awhile I sat in my bedroom and just cried. I talked to a counselor, I worked on my own trauma and fears. But I also used discipline to never let myself fall into despair or into giving up.

In the emergency room, I did not leave his side and I made sure the doctors did not bring needles or medications to him, although I did allow fluids for shock. I made sure they spoke to me (mostly) and not to him as he was coming around. I called in all of the family we had in town (my husband was working out of town). My oldest son, daughter, and niece, ages twenty-two, nineteen, and twenty, met us there. I also had our ten year-old son with us as he had also been riding at the skatepark. He stayed with us the entire time and was allowed to fly in the co-pilot seat on the life-flight because I would not leave him behind. My daughter sat with Aidan and did visualizations right in the e-room as we waited.

Because our small town did not have a pediatric neurologist, or a surgeon for neurology, and there was a very, very small chance that the brain bleed could increase, we decided to take the life-flight to a larger town nearby. It was not a true 'life' flight, in the sense that we all knew Aidan would recover. We transferred to the ambulance, airport, airplane, then a children's hospital the same evening of the injury. Once we got there we met the neurology team and the pediatricians, who already had his records. He was stable, with no worsening symptoms, so we simply slept in the room with him and the nursing staff woke him each hour (in ICU) to check his symptoms. We were transferred out of ICU and into regular care in the hospital the next day (when my husband was able to arrive). The only care they offered there was oxygen (and only because his oxygen monitor was malfunctioning!), checking his blood pressure and monitoring symptoms. He was awake now and fairly clear. He Facetimed his best friends. The hospital staff did their job, but if you do not need surgery or drugs, it is simply a terrible environment to heal in. The constant beeping, 24/7 lights, interruptions, terrible food, lack of fresh air and sunlight all conspire to reduce healing efforts of the body. Aidan was stable and he did not need drugs or surgery, so we decided to check out. They sent us home with a TBI diagnosis and a suggestion we follow-up with our pediatrician, as well as a standard packet about head injury symptoms. The only real recommendation was to rest and bring him to a doctor if symptoms worsened.

Our four hour drive home was rough. The car ride made him nauseous, so we used ice packs and pressure points to reduce that symptom. Once we were home, Aidan was in a semi-conscious state for about four to five days, sleeping around the clock and waking only to eat, drink, and go to the bathroom. When he was awake he was very loopy, having problems discerning reality from his dream-state. His appetite was three-fold normal and his other injuries caused him a lot of pain. He does not remember this week at all, but I do. It was terrifying. However, he only took ibuprofen three times the first week and he refused all other medication (they even offered him morphine in the hospital when he reported a level three on the one to ten scale of pain!). Finally, about 5 days after coming home, Aidan's consciousness returned. He came into our bedroom at about 10 pm (he had been asleep since earlier in the evening) and he said, "Mom, I think I'm finally awake, I feel like myself again". I will never forget those words and that moment! Now we could begin active healing.

We allowed for as much rest as possible, and then built up into a daily checklist of important activities, supplements, and mind-set practices. The first step in this was that we did not use the words 'concussion', 'head injury', or 'TBI' with him at all during the first few weeks of healing. Even the pediatrician was directed, per our request, to not use those words with him during our appointments.

Weird, right?

Not really. We know our son, we knew his triggers and how worried he would be about a head injury. We did not lie. When he asked, we simply said, 'you landed on your face in a bike crash, you have mouth and face injuries, and a separated shoulder - how do you feel?' because that is what happened and his symptoms would tell us what was truly going on. While the label for his problem was 'TBI', *the process of healing in each person is an unknown, the symptoms are ever-changing, and there is no cure or clear path.* So why take on those labels if it won't help him create a powerful mindset for healing? As he became more conscious and aware, he started to ask more questions about his injuries and eventually he came to the conclusion that his brain was affected because of the symptoms he was experiencing. Up until this point, every single, solitary message he had been given was that he was healing beautifully and that he would heal 100%. This allowed him not to worry, and instead focus on what more he could do to heal. He became really engaged in his healing process as the active participant he needed to be to enact virtuous neuroplasticity.

We were relentless in our approach and in turn, so was Aidan. That's how this book was born.

"It is the power of the mind to
be unconquerable."

SENECA

CHAPTER 7

THE PRIMAL PROTOCOL

The Primal Protocol is in no particular order, because each person is a neuro-individual. From varying symptoms to differing goals, healing and supporting the brain is definitely a case-by-case issue. Some people have a beautiful diet, but a super-stressful job, some people have a low-stress life but eat junk food all day, some people work the night-shift. Some people have TBI, some have low energy or early onset Alzheimer's. No one needs the same set of solutions. That said, everyone needs to realign with their biology! It is, of course, always up to you and your care providers what you do, when and how you do it. As always, take precautions, talk to your doctor/s and don't treat this like a medical guide it's an ancestral, evolutionary approach to brain health & injury and you (like we did) are taking your health into your own hands.

I. Get a Primal Mindset

As I explained previously, we must employ the *mind* (your conscious, aware self) to heal the brain and body. You can also employ someone else's mind (or many minds!) to support this effort. The mind is our most powerful tool in this effort. Getting into a mindset of possibility and of healing makes a huge difference. If you don't try anything new, your brain won't even have the chance to respond accordingly.

But what do I mean by 'primal'? Let's imagine our ancestors, and how they could have or would have dealt with TBI. Because modern medicine did not exist, they were dependent on themselves, others and nature to help with their healing. This is also our situation, but we've been cultured to think that we live outside of nature's laws. We don't. We are a biological organism, and our body and brain desperately need what all Earth creatures need: sunlight, clean water, fresh air, the Earth's magnetism, deep sleep, loving relationships and whole, real foods. These make up your path to healing and better performance and are more powerful than almost anything else we can employ. So by 'primal mindset,' I don't just mean you're tough or determined (but that will help!), but you're also clear about what your biology actually needs to survive, heal and thrive.

The new wave of 'functional medicine' is based on an evolutionary approach like this. Functional Medicine (FM) takes into account the whole person and their environment, along with keeping a tether to what a human being is and what they need for baseline health. FM treats the root cause, not the symptoms, and that is what we are doing here as well.

It's the lack of these common evolutionary obligates that leads to DBRS and PDD in the first place, making us less resilient and more prone to neurodegeneration and disease. What is an evolutionary obligate? One great example is this: We humans need two to three hours a day of sunlight to prevent myopia and for optimal eyesight. Sunlight creates dopamine in the eye and helps keep the proper shape of the eye. We are not evolved to be inside at all times. So you are *obligated* to get sunlight. Or at least supplement with Vitamin D if it's winter or circumstances make it difficult to get your required sunlight. Happily, 'getting sun' is usually not an unpleasant task and also offers another benefit; interaction with nature. That is why the evolutionary lens, the ancestral approach, is so critical to regaining brain health. All the effort in the physical therapist's office makes only a tiny dent if the basics are ignored. You can talk to a therapist all day about your depression, but with low vitamin D levels, you aren't addressing a possible cause.

 DO THIS:

- If you are unfamiliar with evolutionary medicine, here are my suggestions:
  - Read this simple blog about evolution and human health, http://mixedmentalarts.online/feisty/
  - Check out The Institute for Functional Medicine or The Ancestral Health Society
  - Read Mark's Daily Apple (an online blog)
  - Check our Chris Kresser's books and website
- If you read these books they can really move your mindset from more-fixed to more-growth:
  - Dr. Norman Doidge, *The Brain's Way of Healing,*
  - JJ Virgin, *Miracle Mindset,*
  - Jocko Willink, *Extreme Ownership*
  - Ryan Holiday, *The Obstacle is the Way*

II. Get Outside

Outside is not a destination, it's actually where humans came to be, it's our home. We are so accustomed to our houses, offices and technology-infused existence we might actually have forgotten this key piece of living! Sunlight, clean water, fresh air, movement and the Earth's magnetism are all found outside. We know that vitamin D deficiency is linked to the chronic fatigue that many people endure after TBI. The absolute best source of vitamin D is the sun on your own skin. Ten minutes in the sun will help your skin cells generate about 10,000 IUs of vitamin D (which is really a secosteroid and not a vitamin). The only other reliable source of vitamin D is in liver, egg yolks and fish.

In National Geographic's extensive article, *This is Your Brain on Nature*, they investigate the new scientific frontier of exploring what happens to the human brain when it is 'exposed' to nature. In one University of Utah study, outdoor education participants showed a fifty percent increase in creative problem-solving after three days in the wilderness. After a fifteen-minute walk in the woods, participants of another study showed a sixteen percent decrease in the stress hormone cortisol, a two percent drop in blood pressure, and a four percent drop in heart rate.

The science is nice, but I will explain the real reason I believe this is critical. In the middle of Aidan's bout with PCS, he received a scholarship from a foundation that supports kids with TBI. We used the money to enroll him in a wilderness education program that met every Friday, all day. We chose that particular program because for a time, we had been responding to his especially bad days by dropping everything and going to a long stretch of sandy beach with great views, just enough driftwood to play on and a relaxed vibe. We would take our canvas pop-up 'cube' that my husband made, blankets, food and just go hang out. Every single time we did this, our son's symptoms would diminish and sometimes disappear. It did not matter what the symptoms were, exposure to more nature helped. So now, each Friday he was spending all day outside, for 7-8 hours - no matter the weather, and learning to build fires, observe animals and find edible plants. Magically, each and every Friday he was feeling good and experiencing no headaches, his depression lifted, he could hike and even run sometimes without feeling foggy.

This reaction to nature-immersion caused me to do my own research and experiments. I am not even an indoorsy-type, but I realized that modern people simply do not spend any significant time outside - unless we work there (like my husband, who is a stonesmith). I started following the work of Katie Bowman, a biomechanist and movement expert. I listened to podcasts about rewilding, which is when people try to regain some of their ancestral heritage to better their health, body mechanics and increased happiness. I read more research, which almost seems like something we should put in the 'duh' category - of course nature is good for you. Then I got into studying screen use, artificial light and nnEMF (see next section). After learning so much and trying different things, our most intensive experiment in this category was, hands down, the fact that we chose to live in a custom-built, canvas pop-up home (tents, very fancy tents) for four months during the summer of 2016. We did this trip when Aidan was seven months post-3rd-TBI. This 24-7 (except for our stops in coffee houses to work and occasional night at a hotel) had profound effects on not only on Aidan's symptoms and general functioning, but all of us had significant positive changes in health and mental functioning.

Below I recommend spending thirty minutes outside everyday, at least ten of that in the sun. This is the minimal, the lowest-level. Ideally, use my 1:1 ratio: One hour on the computer inside equals one hour outside. Good luck! When you put your awareness on this, suddenly the sheer amount of sitting inside, in front of screens gets cast in a whole new light. Pun intended.

 DO THIS:

- Minimal: Spend 30 minutes outside everyday, at least 10 of that in the sun.
- Moderate: Spend 1-2 hours outside, each day doing anything (swimming, walking, gardening, biking)
- Elite: Use my 1:1 ratio. This requires significant lifestyle changes. You may need to build a porch, move part of your office outside, change what kind of work you do, change what you do for 'entertainment', exercise, sports or more.
  - Notes: I realize that for people living in most of the Northern Hemisphere this can be tricky. Winters can be brutal and summers can be too. Make adjustments. I have used Yaktrax and proper boots to be able to take my daily walks in the winter, as well as adjusted my outside time to very early in the morning in very hot and dry environments.

III. Reduce RF and nnEMF Exposure

Non-native electromagnetic frequencies (nnEMFs) and RFs (radio frequencies) are now ubiquitous (everywhere, all-around). Non-native means manmade. We, humans, have our own biomagnetic field (although it is hard to detect) via our own electromagnetic cell processes. The Earth has its own magnetic field. These are all 'native EMFs' and we have evolved to be in harmony with these exposures. In fact, we most likely *need* to be surrounded by and in physical contact with native EMFs to be healthy. It's how we evolved. Consider all the sources of *new* nnEMF and RFs in our lives. The outlets in your walls, all the small appliances we use, all of our computers, televisions, radios, WIFI routers, cell phones, electric lines outside your house, smart meters and cell towers in parks and cities. Our exposure has reached a level never seen before in human history and we have no idea what this is doing and will do to our health. Aligning this technology with biological life just wasn't considered in the developmental phase. It's still not being examined as we rush headlong into 5G and 'smart cities'. Same thing with 'smartphones'.

Consider this study where sixty volunteers spent thirty days sleeping on mats that were either grounded (to the Earth) or ungrounded: Ninety three percent of the grounded participants slept better, eighty two percent had less muscle stiffness and pain and seventy four percent experienced elimination of chronic pain. Check the references section (Elizabeth, 2017) for a list of 34 additional scientific studies showing adverse health effects from exposure to WIFI. The basic rules for lessening nnEMF exposure are:

- Turn off your WIFI at night, or hardwire computers at home
- Do not place your bed near unused outlets, and/or use EMI filters that plug into the outlet
- Do not carry your cellphone on your body (each cell phone has the recommendations listed somewhere in the general info on the phone, ranges vary)
- Do not put a cellphone up to your head when talking (use earbuds, or air tubes)

- Do not place your laptop on your lap or body
- Turn off things you are not using (lights, computers, phones, radios, etc)

 DO THIS:

- Unplug your WIFI at night or hardwire your home/office
- Use a protective carrying device (like Safesleeve products) to reduce exposure from cell phones, tablets and laptop

IV. Reduce Screen Time & Artificial Light

The average American child spends about seven hours per day on the screen through use of computers, phones, tablets, and television. For adults, it's an average of ten hours. If you spend eight hours sleeping, then ten hours on the screen, that leaves you six hours for life. Only six hours for nature, relationships, eating, exercise and fun. And I just told you to spend two of that six outside. Just in practical terms, this is a silly state of affairs, but for your brain it's deleterious. Your brain hates screen time! Dr. Dunckley, who writes for *Psychology Today*, says that many children may have electronic screen syndrome (ESS - I know, another 'disease', but again, I use these phrases as a catch-all, an easy way to translate complicated ideas or symptoms) and suffer impulsiveness, moodiness and problems with sleep due to overuse of electronic screens. Sadly, addiction (I said your brain hated screen time, I didn't say it couldn't be addicted) to the internet and phone is a thing, and there are quite a few studies showing physical and electrical damage such as gray matter atrophy, loss of white matter integrity, cravings, impaired cognitive function to the brain from this very anti-primal behavior. For a brain that is healing, this is a huge no-no. For a healthy brain, this is a great way to wear it out and down. There are no standards for what would be ideal because again, we haven't studied the enormous impact of this new behavior, but less is probably more in this case.

One reason screentime is so damaging is because it automatically exposes us to lots and lots of artificial light in the blue and green spectrum. There is (luckily) quite a bit of solid research about how this overexposure interrupts sleep, disrupts hormone regulation and even has connections to some cancers. We evolved to be exposed to full-spectrum, bright light during the day, and darkness at night. In fact, this is a critical component of our biology. Light is the conductor of our circadian rhythm and that biological rhythm is the foundation upon which our health rests.

Finally, be aware it's not just screens. All those new LED bulbs we are using also generally fall in the blue/green spectrum.

 DO THIS:

- Track your screen time and then reduce it
- Use Flux, Screenshader, Night Watch or other apps and programs that will automatically cut down the blue and green spectrum during nighttime use of screens
- Buy blue-blocking glasses for use during nighttime activities where you are being exposed to a lot of artificial light
- Buy full-spectrum lights, or better yet, use only amber lights at night

Because we all probably overuse our internet connection, phones, tablets, TV, laptop and games; here are alternatives to the screen:

- Social time (hang out with people you like and love)
- Reading (if you can, and if you can't you need to retrain your brain to do this - start with magazines, or bigger print books)
- Writing (another skill to work on)
- Board and card games (great for hand-eye coordination, as well as getting the brain to think differently)
- Art (any kind, whatever you can manage - pencils, watercolors, clay - also great for the healing brain)
- Yoga or any movement challenges balance and strength
- Walking (walking may be the single-most unused brain healing technique ever!!!)
- Swimming
- Cooking (it's a creative and novel activity every single time)
- Building, sewing, leather-working (even tinker toys or erector sets can be super helpful)
- Music - Make it, play it, listen to it
- There is much, much more - engage in LIFE

V. Rest

I am not even going to cite any science here. Your brain needs rest to recover. While you sleep the brain is really, really busy getting things cleaned up and organized. You must let it do this. It's very common after head injury for the injured person to sleep a lot. This is critical! It's one reason college students do not recover as quickly from head injury compared the rest of the population. They study too much and sleep too little.

Oh wait! That's everyone, not just college students. So many of us are working too hard, too many hours, and sacrificing sleep to watch a movie late at night. Twenty percent of Americans report getting less than six hours of sleep a night. This causes a cascade of emotional and physical problems, and it also increases highway and driving deaths. It's a serious, serious issue.

I know for many of us, getting more sleep may seem impossible. In our culture we press on, push forward and try to continue with life no matter what. In the end, the result of ignoring what your brain needs is low function, brain fog, weight gain, emotional issues, Post Concussion Syndrome (PCS) and more - none of it good!

When my son suffered that third injury, I had to quit my full-time job and my PhD program. I ended up homeschooling him so he could keep up with his grade level but not have to endure eight hours in the school environment which is loud, brightly lit and stressful. Critically, being out of school he could also sleep as much as his body needed.

Was this convenient? No, but we figured it out anyway. We had to prioritize sleep, even if our modern world didn't.

Since learning so much about the brain, I've stopped using an alarm clock and have no electronics in my room at all. I also use blackout curtains. I sleep deeply. In the winter I get about ten hours of sleep (no I am not kidding!) and in the summer, I get about eight hours because I let my sleep cycle 'just happen' and this is what it's evolved into.

DO THIS:

- Stop using the screen one hour before you go to sleep
- Add 30 minutes to your sleep schedule (go to bed earlier, get up later)
- Darken your sleeping room
- Remove most, if not all, electronics from your bedroom
- Use a fan or white noise to distract from jarring sounds
- Keep your sleeping room as cool as you can (humans sleep better when it's a little colder)
- Do not sleep with your phone next to your body or head! Use a real alarm clock if you must

VI. Social Support

Humans are an interdependent species. We can't truly survive on our own, and it's not only about survival. Social support and relationships have a huge effect on your health and your brain, *even bigger than diet*. Yes, relationships are more powerful than what you eat and that's pretty damn powerful! If you are isolated or surrounded by toxic emotions, you'll suffer for it. Your brain health will suffer. We are a socially intelligent and sensitive species, so it's critical to respect that fact, and actively set up a social life that helps make you healthy.

Have you heard of the Roseto Effect? Roseto, Pennsylvania was an Italian settlement with an unusually low rate of heart attacks. Doctors studied the entire village from 1954 - 1961, and even though the population had all the high-risk factors for heart disease, during that time no heart attacks occured. They then did a 50 year study comparing Roesto to nearby Bangor and determined that is was the

Italian-style social structure that was health-protective to members of the community. The people of Roseto smoked, ate fried sausages and drank wine like crazy with no increase of disease. Why? The relationships in their village were very close, they had their own social safety net and the people knew they could depend on each other.

 DO THIS:

- Eat dinner, with people you like/love, just about every night.
- If you have one or more toxic relationships, especially where abuse is occurring, take action. These relationships wear down our immunity and stress out our brain. Whether it's quitting a job, getting into counseling with a spouse or ditching a toxic friend, you need to protect yourself and your health.
- Set up time with friends and family to just hang out. Go to a park or a coffee house, talk, read books out loud, play games, and do these activities face-to-face. Real social engagement is great for us!
- If you don't have a strong network or need to make connections, try asking people at your church, workplace or other community and social groups to run errands, take you to appointments, grocery shop or walk with you – people want to be social and connect and they also like helping others.
- If your activities are reduced, you may find yourself more isolated. You can also listen to podcasts, books on tape (like Audible) or play music. This can lessen the effects of loneliness. Additionally, apps like Apple's Facetime or Skype can provide face-to-face conversations with people who are far away.

VII. What to Eat/Nutrition

Here we go. Food is so tribalized right now. You've got your Vegan Tribe, the Paleo Cavepeople, the Clean-Eaters, the Keto Clan, the Grain Brain Society, the Bulletproof Dynasty and the Food Allergy Horde.

You've got lectins and leptin and glucose metabolism and calories-in/calories-out, or calories don't matter. You've got the GMO-free, no-RoundUp Society and the Avoiding Mold Club.

What in the hell are you going to do?

Food is medicine - it *is* important. Here are my thoughts on diet:

First things first. Make sure your food is food and not some chemical composition masquerading as food.

Know that low carbohydrate, high-fat (LCHF) diets have been used since the 1920s to treat people with seizures and this is a common recommendation for people with brain injury. There are many versions of this type of eating; LCHF, nutritional ketosis, a modified Atkins diet and the low glycemic index treatment (LGIT). If you're unfamiliar with these, the premise is simple - to eat significantly less carbohydrates (grains, fruits, veggies, sugars) and higher healthy fat, with a moderate protein intake.

This particular pathway helps the brain because of something called ketones. Ketones are produced by the liver, when the body has run out of sugars (glucose) to burn. They are our alternative energy source, and our ability to run on this energy source protects humans during periods of starvation. Breastfed babies are 'in ketosis' much of the time. Mild ketosis has been proven to have therapeutic effects on the brain in multiple studies and some research indicates the brain seems to be more efficient when it's running on ketones!

There are three paths to ketosis. One is to eat a nutritional ketosis diet. The second (most recent) path is to supplement with exogenous ketones, which are ketones made in a lab that you can drink. Finally, you can try intermittent fasting.

I highly suggest working with a nutritionist or nutritional coach.

If it's for your child, definitely seek medical guidance! You can buy all kinds of exogenous ketones online now, but I recommend doing your research. If you choose to intermittent fast, follow a guide (many are available online) and talk to your doctor.

Not everyone is a good candidate for these kinds of nutritional interventions.

At the very least, however, you must stop eating sugar. I'm sorry, but it's true! Your brain is very sensitive to the overabundance of sugars in the S.A.D. (standard American diet) and you will only delay healing if you are dumping unnecessary sugars into your belly.

Additionally, there is a decent body of research showing that eliminating wheat, if not most grains, has benefits for the brain as well. The book, *Grain Brain* by Dr. Perlmutter, explains this in detail. For instance, most people have some gluten-sensitivity (with or without celiac being present). Gluten is a protein found in wheat, barley and rye. This reactivity to gluten increases the production of inflammatory cytokines that are known to be neurodegenerative.

I also recommend eating as much organic, whole, real food as possible. Read labels and avoid the common chemicals and additives that are in pre-packaged food. Learn to cook! You'll save money, have fun and eat better.

If you change your diet, remember that there are serious consequences to doing 'keto' incorrectly by not taking enough magnesium, consuming too little calories, eating way too much fat, avoiding all animal products or eliminating any large group of foods. Use your common-sense and talk to someone knowledgeable about it.

If you are on medications or have seizures or serious physical ailments, you must, must, must get professional help with this!

I am not a doctor and I do not play one on television, so please get help with your nutrition.

 DO THIS:

- Reduce or eliminate your processed sugar intake. Hint: In my opinion, it's easier to quit sugar all-out than to just allow so much here and there or have 'cheat days'.
- Try going gluten-free (and maybe grain free). Give yourself a solid 30-60 days of a strict no-gluten diet. Most people have a very positive reaction to this test, including reduced depression, less headaches, weight loss and more mental clarity.
- Michael Pollan, author of the *Omnivore's Dilemma*, says, "Eat food, not too much, mostly plants". I love this. Concentrate on food that food, not a chemical copy of food, don't overeat and eat a lot of plants.
  - Most of my plates look like this: A bunch of greens, a little fruit, maybe some squash or sweet potatoes, a few nuts/seeds, some well-sourced protein and that's it. Most of it is organic, pasture-raised, as local as I can get it. I do my best with what I can access.
  - I (and my whole family) never, ever eat or serve these things: Chemicals of any kind, food coloring, processed fats (i.e. margarine), sugar of all kinds, soda, candy or pre-baked goods (i.e. muffins)

VIII. Supplements

There are so many supplements, herbs and compounds that are recommended by thousands of various practitioners from Chinese medicine doctors to chiropractors. In the next section, I try to list anything that has some reasonable science or solid anecdotal support but if you want my quick take, *and most people do*, here is what I recommend:

 DO THIS:

- Fish oil (purified, high-quality, high DHA)
- Lion's Mane (mushroom)
- NAC (n-acetyl cysteine)
- Turmeric or ginger (fresh or in capsules)

We can do something, many things, for our brain. Whether it's healing it, getting more out of it or protecting it from disease. Drop the cultural message that we can't heal - we can. Forget limitations. Forget weakness. Apply your will and intelligence and you can solve anything. We are meant to feel amazing, to be clear and experience joy. Give it a shot.

IX. Exercise and Movement

Regular exercise improves memory, protects thinking skills, increases the size of the hippocampus in the brain and increases brain-derived neurotrophic factor (BDNF). Exercise reduces inflammation and insulin resistance. People who move a lot have a brain that is higher in volume (heavier) and they have tighter and more neural connections. One hour, twice a week is enough to make changes in the brain and that's nothing. Walking, yoga, dancing, swimming - it doesn't matter. Do what you enjoy, just move.

PS - Exercise will also improve your mood. A lot.

 DO THIS:

- I really recommend that you walk outside each and every day (when it's possible). This habit hits multiple targets with one easy and pleasurable activity! You need the nature, the sun, vitamin D, movement, varied terrain and socializing. A regular walk will accomplish that and more. 30 minutes, outside, daily. More if you can. Humans are walking/running machines and without out this activity our brian suffers and walking in nature is healing on many levels.

"Happiness is not a matter of intensity, but of balance, order, rhythm and harmony."

THOMAS MERTON

CHAPTER 8

THE HORMONE SWITCH

From glucagon to ghrelin, enkephalin to insulin and testosterone to estrogen, our entire body is modulated by hormones. How we experience pain and regulate blood sugar is informed and regulated by hormones. We have glands and organs in our bodies that make all these hormones; the ovaries, your fat tissue and even your heart create various substances that are essential to daily functioning. This system is overseen by two master glands in the brain. You knew I was getting to the brain, right? The hypothalamus and the pituitary glands work together and both regulate (through very complicated methods) all the functions of your sex organs, growth, energy, hunger, circadian rhythms and much, much more.

Would you be surprised if I told you that any injury to the brain (chemical, addiction, concussion, TBI, acquired brain injury [ABI], etc) can cause significant hormone deficiencies even years after the injury? I was certainly surprised to learn this! Approximately fifty to seventy percent of people with brain injury will experience transitional hormone deficiency that seems to be caused by pituitary malfunction. Worse than that, over fifty percent of people will experience these deficiencies *one year* or more post-injury. People with endocrine (hormone) dysregulation experience problems ranging from unexplained fatigue to higher rates of depression, post-concussion syndrome that will not resolve, PCOS (polycystic ovarian syndrome) and issues with blood-sugar regulation.

Dr. Mark L. Gordon of the Millenium TBI Project (he also works with the Warrior Angels Foundation) is an expert in this subject and in treating TBI via hormone replacement. He and his colleagues have worked extensively with the military using this approach successfully. When growth hormone, testosterone, estrogen, progesterone, thyroid and cortisol are too low or too high the symptoms are numerous and nearly the whole body is affected. Usually when we think of 'T-levels' - this is what the men in my family call testosterone - we only think of sex or aggression. However, sex steroid hormones (like estrogen and progesterone) are actually made from cholesterol and they easily cross through the blood-brain barrier. Once inside the central nervous system (CNS), the hormones act on receptor targets and trigger changes, like adjusting neurotransmitter levels, which affects both the brain structures and various functions. So it's not all about sex or muscles.

So how do you know if something in your endocrine system is off? Simple: Symptoms and/or testing. Low testosterone causes low sex-drive, hair loss, muscle-mass loss and depression (among other symptoms). Low cortisol can also include depression and additionally; muscle weakness, headaches, low-back pain, nausea, anxiety and insomnia. Low estrogen can produce night sweats, insomnia and weight gain. Allendocrine disruption affects the mood. It just goes on and on. But hormone dysregulation is tied to brain injury (i.e. brain injury of any kind can lead to low levels of critical hormones) and conversely, low hormone levels can lead to brain malfunctions (i.e. like when estrogen drops off in menopause, many women have brain fog and forgetfulness).

Hormones can be affected by many environmental factors, not just injury. Autoimmune diseases and stress can cause changes in hormone secretion and uptake. Endocrine disrupting chemicals (EDCs) like certain pesticides, lead, PCBs, dioxins, parabens and anti-bacterial chemicals all cause problems with the human hormone system. There are even foods that mimic estrogen (known as estrogenic compounds) like soy and flax seeds that can cause issues, especially for boys and men. And for those who are newer marijuana users, the plant appears to have a suppressive effect on the sex hormones, growth hormone and prolactin, but this seems to decline over time as tolerance is built.

This is all bad enough for adults, but for kids, it's especially scary.

Dr. Gordon states in his article, *Traumatic Brain Injury – Hormonal Dysfunction Syndrome; "The Stealth Syndrome"*, that "it is extremely important to give all prepubescent children who have sustained a head injury a total hormone assessment, because that head injury may cause pTBI-HDS [post Traumatic Brain Injury-Hormone Deficiency Syndrome], which could cause a whole range of problems, including short stature, personality changes, functional disability, and problems with language skills and school skills".

Ok, so what do we do? In this case, I actually advise something not very 'primal' - testing. You can somewhat reliably test for hormones using some pretty simple blood and/or saliva tests. Because everyone has a different kind of health insurance, doctor and scenario, I can't say what you should do exactly. Ideally, you would be working with a great functional medicine doctor and he/she would order the labs for you and help you interpret them and then decide on a pathway forward. Ha! Most people will not have those options. If not, you can go through a regular doctor and examine the tests yourself. Or you can order the labs on your own and biohack your own way through this. Life Extension and Everlywell are but two companies of many that offer one-off testing direct to the consumer (in this case that's us!).

That said, you don't have to test. Symptoms are a great illuminator. This is your path, your healing journey and the decisions are yours.

So what to do once you realize (or suspect) you've got HDS (Hormone Deficiency Syndrome)? Again, it depends. Some people get hormone replacement therapy (HRT) through a doctor or clinic. I would call this tool the heavy hammer. Save it for last, in case other, lower-level efforts do not work. Most people will benefit from the lifestyle and nutrition suggestions I make in the Primal Protocol, but there *are* specific supplements, compounds and behaviors that will assist the endocrine system. My suggestions follow:

Red Light Therapy

Red light therapy, also known as low-level laser therapy (LLLT), has been used for a long time to assist with wound healing and to reduce skin ageing. Research has demonstrated that applying red light to the body will increase collagen, stimulate the immune system, activate the lymph system, increase production of ATP, reduce joint pain, reduce depression symptoms and increase blood flow. Recently, whole-body red light therapy has been used as a treatment for diabetes, and is used in some clinics as therapy for brain injury. Red light was shown in one study to reduce hypothyroidism in forty five participants. Diabetes and hypothyroidism are endocrine disorders. I think this therapy is cutting-edge and we will see more and more light therapy solutions coming to the forefront of modern medicine. Until then, there are clinics that offer red light therapy and there are multiple devices (from inexpensive to very expensive) available for home use. Clinics are offering intranasal red light therapy in conjunction with other treatments to reduce the symptoms of Parkinson's as well. There are no known side-effects with light therapy.

Supplementation

Certain minerals and vitamins are critical for hormone production. You can assist your body's attempts to get back into balance by making sure you get enough:

- Magnesium
- Selenium
- Zinc
- Vitamin K2
- Vitamin D
- Cholesterol

Nutritional Support

Eating enough protein and fat is critical to hormone balance and because some of the major players (i.e. testosterone, Vitamin D and bile salts) are derived and delivered via cholesterol, these proteins and fats need to be animal-based. Additionally, sugar is not a friend to the hormone system. Like I said, reduce, if not eliminate sugars from your diet to optimize your body's ability to stay in balance and increase the hormones you need. These foods in particular are amazing for endocrine health:

- Avocados
- Broccoli
- Bone Broth
- Coconut (oil, meat, flaked)
- Eggs
- Wild Fish
- Grass-Fed Whey

Targeted Exercise

Moving your body is important (crucial!), but if you want to trigger growth hormone and testosterone, certain types of exercise are better than others.

- HIIT (high intensity interval training) has been clearly shown to boost testosterone levels when compared to 'steady state exercise'.
- Sprinting will also create the same endocrine response. It doesn't have to be running either (which can be rough for

those who have head injury, PCS or headaches/migraines). You can use a rowing machine or exercise/real bike as well.

- Weight lifting will trigger growth hormone and testosterone (as well as a ton of other neurochemicals that are beneficial).

Lifestyle Changes

- Get sunlight! The best form of vitamin D comes from the sun. You need plenty of sunlight for your brain's glands to send all the right signals to your testes, ovaries and adrenal glands.
- Reduce stress! Stress (toxic, unending, chronic) is a hormone killer. Make lifestyle changes to bring more harmony into your life. Learn to meditate, do yoga or exercise in order to modulate your body's response to stress.
- Sleep! We are a nation of sleep-deprived people. Sleep is critical to brain health, and your two master glands in there need the rest as well. Clean up your sleep hygiene (no electronics before bed, get the TV out of the bedroom, don't sleep with your phone, make your room dark and cool) and get to bed earlier to start acclimating yourself to a real circadian clock.

Herbs

Herbs and plants like vitex, cinnamon, astragalus, holy basil, clary sage, ashwagandha, shilajit, maca, red raspberry, milk thistle, oat straw, black cohosh, saw palmetto (and that's just a short list) can all help assist the endocrine system. There are probably thousands of plants that have specific effects on the hormone system (and thus, the brain).

Additionally, there are many books devoted to herbs and their uses and there are professionals called herbalists who can help you navigate the diverse world of plants.

I hit on each of these topics in the Primal Protocol, as they are all interwoven into multiple facets of brain health. It's impossible to just unwind hormones from the body or brain, it all works together.

However, the brain and endocrine system are tightly wired together and I've found that many people benefit from simply adding zinc and/or vitamin D to their supplement regime or or from doing intranasal red light therapy.

"You have power over your mind –
not outside events. Realize this, and
you will find strength."

MARCUS AURELIUS

CHAPTER 9

CHILD BRAIN HEALTH, WOMEN'S BRAIN HEALTH & THE MILITARY

The Importance of Child Brain Health

There are two specific issues regarding kids and brain health that are important to understand. One is brain injury and how it affects future brain health, and the other is protecting brain health in kids who are not injured.

When children sustain brain injuries they are more likely to suffer from anxiety, depression, Parkinson's Disease (in the future), metabolic changes, DNA damage and increased oxidative stress over their lifetime, not just post-injury. These are just the topics that have been studied. We really don't know exactly what other issues brain injury in childhood may cause later in life at this point. Because of this very serious risk, I believe that it's important to continue to treat any negative brain symptoms, even if it takes years, until they are cleared (if possible, as much as possible).

Bringing the brain back into balance and full health should confer protection from problems later in life. Although, no one is really studying that either, as we are just emerging from a paradigm where the belief was that healing is limited by scope and time. The research on neuroplasticity proves this isn't true - improving brain health and performance is possible all the time, at any time, throughout the lifespan.

Children who suffer multiple or grievous head injuries might need to make permanent changes to lifestyle that include

- reduced chemical exposure
- a stricter diet regime
- specific exercise
- stress-reduction techniques
- reduced exposure to RF and nMFs
- psychological support

Whatever the trade is, it's worth it to avoid the later-in-life brain disease, Parkinson's, that currently affects five million people. That number is expected to exceed fourteen million cases by 2050. Parkinson's Disease affects about 60,000 Americans each year. CTE (chronic traumatic encephalopathy) is probably the scariest result of repeated head trauma. Sports that have high impact, like football, hockey and boxing, are definitely connected to CTE, but it can occur in situations where blast trauma occurs or with domestic abuse as well. New diagnostic techniques are emerging as this book goes to print. Symptoms of CTE include memory loss, confusion, personality disorders, suicidal behavior, depression and erratic behavior.

Aside from brain injury, we need to talk about kids' brain health in general. Modern children are exposed to a host of neurotoxic situations.

With poor nutrition, too much sugar, noise pollution, air and water pollution, chemical exposure, constant exposure to artificial light, too much time spent indoors, emotional stress and over-exposure to WIFI and RFs (radio-frequencies from phones), our kids are in real danger of chronic, low brain health - diminishment. If a child has low vitamin D levels, and many do, this affects brain health and development, as do low zinc levels or problems with gut bacteria. Making sure children have great nutrition is critical, as is controlling their electronic environment, encouraging time spent outside and making sure they have a lifestyle that includes moving their body. In this way, securing a healthy brain for the future is possible.

There is No Unisex Brain - Women's Brain Health

The newest research reveals information about women's brain health that is concerning at the very least. Female athletes appear to take twice as long as their male counterparts to heal from concussion. They also sustain higher rates of head injury in general. Women's smaller necks might make them more prone to suffer a head injury in the first place. Women also have higher rates of glucose metabolism which impacts brain healing negatively as well. Finally, the female menstrual cycle seems to affect brain health and healing, as hormones play a critical role in brain health (as I just mentioned in Chapter 8). For instance, progesterone is protective to the brain and supportive to the healing process. Yet at certain times during a woman's cycle, progesterone drops rapidly and may slow the brain's ability to heal.

While women athletes are more likely than their male counterparts to report head injury to coaches and medical personnel, there is a group of women almost utterly ignored and who rarely report injury; victims of domestic violence. Estimates are that as many as twenty million women each year might have TBI caused by domestic violence.

That would be six percent of the entire U.S. population. Additionally, most women are not only not talking about it, they are not screened in emergency rooms or shelters. This is another unique component of the female experience (currently) that needs to be considered by professionals and women themselves as they navigate these tough situations.

For the general population, we can use information about head injury to steer a path to better brain health and performance. If women have cyclical drops in critical hormones - and their brain is particularly sensitive during the postpartum and menopause period - they may need additional support to improve general performance and might be more at risk for symptoms that seem to have no origin but are actually emanating from the brain. My anecdotal experience with many female clients is that they are often misdiagnosed with 'psychological' issues and not screened for brain problems leading to drawn-out recoveries and a lot of frustration and suffering. Remember WNL? This is especially true for women. In fact, it smacks of a time when women were diagnosed with things like 'hysteria'.

Finally, women (in multiple areas of medicine) have not been included in many studies on brain injury, health and function. Even when researchers use mice and rats, the models are often male. That means that our understanding of the differences between male and female brain injury are really just in the beginning stages!

Military Injuries and Factors

Military service members also have unique circumstances. Sometimes called the 'signature injury' of the Iraq and Afghanistan wars, TBI is very (very!) prevalent in the military. Head injury can be caused by blast injuries (known as bTBI and often caused by IEDs), vehicle and motorcycle accidents and falls. There are other jobs in the military that lead to more exposure and risk as well. For instance, repetitive shooting drills can increase exposure to lead, which is a known neurotoxin. There are so many jobs in the military and all carry varying levels of risk- I cannot cover them all here.

One massively important issue is suicide. In any situation for any person, a head injury leads to a three-fold higher risk for suicide. The high suicide rate in the military is a well-known problem. With thirty suicides for every 100,000 service members, the military rate is much higher than the general population rate of twelve for every 100,000 (which is still very high!). Add a head or chemical-induced brain injury to the military scenario, and the risk for suicide is extremely high.

Because our culture, including the medical culture, still believes there isn't much you can do for head injury, it's critical to get the Primal Brain message out to the military. There are many paths to healing the brain! It's important for service members and veterans to acquire a care coordinator and to seek more than the standard Western medical model for healing. There are no pharmaceuticals that can cure most brain issues at this point. Each and every drug is to treat symptomology, and many drugs are harmful to brain health. Unless there is bleeding in the brain or a mass, generally, there is no surgery procedure for head trauma that happened in the past. Physical therapy and cognitive behavior therapy (psychotherapy) are both helpful in healing brain injury and trauma, but there is so much more to do! There are many independent groups and advocates that offer great resources and support to current and former military personnel, as well as non-profits that have special services. It's worth looking outside the standard to find solutions.

"Healing is a matter of time,
but it is sometimes also a matter
of opportunity."

HIPPOCRATES

CHAPTER 10

NOOTROPIC NUTRACEUTICALS

Nootropic nutraceuticals - supplements or functional foods that enhance cognitive functions like intelligence, memory, and focus - are a burgeoning new industry within the supplement market. We will be seeing more and more of these products in addition to the original nootropics (pronounced 'no-eh-tropics'), which are a class of pharmaceuticals drugs. The word was coined by Romanian psychologist and chemist, Dr. Corneliu E. Giurgea, who synthesized the first nootropic, *piracetam*, over fifty years ago. I am not endorsing any of these (drugs, herbs, etc.) and there are many products I'm not aware of or have no experience with. I don't use myself or family members as guinea pigs, so I just don't have encyclopedic knowledge at this time. But it's worth looking into!

Below is an A-Z list of various remedies I've researched, crowd-sourced or tried. These are in alphabetical order, not by importance. This guide is NOT medical advice! This guide is not comprehensive! You should do your own research or have your care provider, care coordinator or at least a family member research and assist with further investigation before you jump into using any nootropics.

Arnica Montana (external and internal)

Arnica is a plant of the daisy family that bears yellow flowers. One of the most used homeopathic (a style of medicine using minute doses of natural substances) medicines, often for bruising and contusions, and great for initial healing.

Artichoke Extract

This is currently being marketed as a nootropic. Studies show some benefit in glucose metabolism when participants were taking artichoke extract. Anything that helps with glucose metabolism will have at least a small benefit to the brain.

Ashwagandha

Ashwagandha, an Indian herb, has been shown to increase myelin levels in the nervous system. It also is beneficial to the thyroid and adrenal glands and can help reduce cortisol (our stress hormone). It's also helpful in stabilizing blood sugar, which is important to the brain.

Astaxanthin

Astaxanthin is a keto-carotenoid. It belongs to a larger class of chemical compounds known as terpenes. Naturally derived from algae, there are also synthetic versions (we used the actual plant). It has been shown to reduce symptoms in brain injury.

B Vitamins

B vitamins are a class of water-soluble vitamins that play important roles in cell metabolism. Though these vitamins share similar names, research shows that they are chemically distinct vitamins that often coexist in the same foods. Research shows these can improve sensorimotor function, help elevate mood and increase energy.

Bacopa

Bacopa is an aquatic plant that needs to be taken with food (as some people will have an upset stomach from taking it alone). In scientific studies it's been shown to improve cognition by reducing anxiety. It promotes neuro-communication and interacts with dopamine and serotonin.

Bone Broth

This isn't a fad, it's what your Grandma used to make - it's called soup. Loaded with minerals, collagen and more good stuff it will soothe and heal the digestive tract and help regulate blood sugar while delivering important nutrients to your brain.

Cat's Claw

Cat's Claw is an herb that fights brain inflammation and oxidative stress. It also Promotes healthy cerebral circulation and can help "dissolve" amyloid plaques that are associated with brain degeneration.

CBD Oil

Cannabidiol is a non psychoactive (meaning you cannot get high from it) constituent of the marijuana plant. Available in states where cannabis is legal either medically or recreationally, CBD oil has a well-earned reputation as friend to the brain. From reducing damage just post-TBI to helping people heal from stroke to stopping medication-resistant seizures, CBD holds promise as a true miracle worker for the brain. My only caveat: I prefer to use whole plant, as this confer the most the plant has to offer. A CBD oil that has the proper balance THC might give you some 'sensations', but in my book (this is my book after all!) is a better treatment.

Cedar oil (patchouli, vetiver, myrrh, frankincense, sandalwood)

These essential oils have sesquiterpenes, which help increase oxygen delivery to the brain (by up to 28%). They smell wonderful and can be used in conjunction with meditation or breathing exercising. NOT topically - to be diffused into the air only.

Coenzyme Q10

This is an important oil-soluble, vitamin-like substance found in your mitochondria that helps create energy.

D3 & K2

Vitamin D refers to a group of fat-soluble secosteroids responsible for enhancing intestinal absorption of calcium, iron, magnesium, phosphate and zinc. Vitamin K refers to a group of structurally similar, fat-soluble vitamins the human body needs for complete synthesis of certain proteins that are required for blood coagulation. Both vitamin D and K are critical in reducing oxidative stress and inflammation. Vitamin D also increases absorption of minerals in the intestinal tract. It's also shown to be helpful in healing brain injury.

DHA (Omega 3 Fatty Acids)

Docosahexaenoic acid is an omega-3 fatty acid that is a primary structural component of the human brain, cerebral cortex, skin, sperm, testicles and retina. DHA decreases cellular injury and inflammation, especially in the brain. In fact, I cannot overstate the need for more Omega 3's in the human diet. It's just critical. A MUST.

Epsom Salt Baths (and/or magnesium supplements)

Epsom salt is magnesium sulfate and in some studies it has been shown to influence improvement on the Glasgow Outcome Scale (this scale categorizes brain injured patients by severity). It is also a common folk treatment for people with concussion and head injury. Baths are not only relaxing, but the healing brain needs magnesium.

Ginkgo Biloba

The leaves from the Ginkgo tree (one of the oldest tree species on the planet) are used to manage dementia, anxiety, headache, ringing ears, low blood flow to the brain, and difficulty concentrating. It has been used for thousands of years.

HRT (Hormone Replacement Therapy)

It's been repeatedly demonstrated that hormones are impacted by brain injury of any kind. Our hormones are deeply affected by our general health and exposure to chemicals in everyday life- it's a smart choice to get a hormone panel and make sure nothing is really out of whack. You can use a service like Everlywell or see your doctor to get labs drawn.

Iodine

Iodine is a key mineral that supports thyroid function. Low thyroid hormone impairs the production of myelin and the process of myelination.

Iron

Iron is critical in the production of ATP (the energy in our cells). It's cheap and smart to get your levels checked and supplement if needed.

Lion's Mane (Mushrooms)

Hericium erinaceus is an edible and medicinal mushroom belonging to the tooth fungus group. Native to North America, Europe and Asia it can be identified by its long spines. Lion's Mane reduces oxidative stress and improves cognitive function even if brain injury already happened. An absolute essential in our plan.

Lithium

Lithium is an essential mineral, not just a treatment for bipolar disorder. Lithium orotate is available over-the-counter and can be taken to help restore brain health (depending on symptoms) because it helps in the remyelination process.

MCT Oil/Coconut Oil

MCT simply stands for medium chain triglycerides (a type of fat), as opposed to long chain triglycerides (LCT), which are found in most foods. MCT is comprised of primarily caprylic and capric fatty acids, and is a light-yellow, odorless, translucent liquid at room temperature. MCT oil occurs naturally in coconut oil and other foods.

Melatonin

Most know of this as the sleep hormone. When we sleep we produce oligodendrocyte precursor cells (OPCs). The formation of these cells doubles while we sleep (according to studies on mice) and they assist in myelination. Myelin is a fatty, white substance that wraps around the end of many nerve cells insulating them and increasing the speed at which they send electrical signals. Myelin is critical to brain health. Without proper amounts of melatonin produced in the brain, we don't/won't sleep well. You can take over-the-counter melatonin or engage in great sleep hygiene (no screens before bed, cool your room down, unplug the WIFI, blackout your room, etc).

Mulberry Leaf

In studies on rats, Mulberry Leaf protected the brain against neuroinflammation and oxidative stress when the brain was exposed to glyphosate (the herbicide in RoundUp).

NAC (N-Acetyl Cysteine)

One study showed 'significant behavioral recovery' using NAC after TBI in rats. NAC has also been proven to reduce cerebral inflammation following TBI. It's also been shown to increase mitochondrial function when administered immediately post-injury. Basically, this should be administered in every emergency with all TBI patients. A critical component we used immediately after injury.

Phosphatidylserine

This is a fat-soluble amino acid that has been shown to improve attention and memory. Even the FDA says that is may slow cognitive decline and reduce the risk of dementia.

Pregnenolone

Pregnenolone is a precursor all the other steroid hormones like DHEA, progesterone, testosterone, estrogen and cortisol. It can enhance memory and reduce fatigue. We make our own, but if your levels are off you can supplement with it via over-the-counter products.

Probiotics (Low-Histamine)

The brain and gut have an intimate relationship based on which colonies of bacteria are thriving and which ones are not. You truly cannot heal the brain without healing the gut. It is critical to brain health to restore and improve the gut biome! Histamine reducing probiotics are best, as they reduce inflammation throughout the body.

Book: Brain Maker by Dr. Perlmutter

Salt

Salt is another critical nutrient that assists in almost every function in the body. Not enough sat will make it harder to sleep, make things difficult for your thyroid gland and mess with your blood pressure.

Saturated Fat

Fat-phobia is over. You need cholesterol to make hormones (like testosterone) and vitamin D. Grass-fed butter, egg yolks and beef liver are great choices.

Turmeric (or Ginger or both)

Is a bright yellow root of the plant, Turmeric, a member of the ginger family (commonly used in curry, although not spicy). Turmeric has antifungal and antibiotic properties, but is known for its anti-inflammatory effect on the whole body. Research supports the possible use for brain injury recovery.

Vitamin C

Collagen is critical to the production of myelin and collagen synthesis is dependent on vitamin c, which is cheap and easy to find. You can also eat more green leafy veggies, citrus fruits, tomatoes and berries.

Zinc

A deficiency in zinc can impair brain function in both children and adults. Zinc is a trace mineral that assists in hundreds of enzymatic reactions in the body, including helping neurotransmitters. It is estimated that two billion people in the world are deficient in zinc.

"Time is the scarcest resource and unless it is managed, nothing else can be managed."

PETER DRUCKER

CHAPTER II

TREATMENTS AND RESOURCES

Many people with TBI, brain fog or other impediments to brain health attempt to include other treatments that are not on Western medical model's radar. Hyperbaric oxygen treatment, chiropractic, massage therapy, acupuncture, Chinese herbs, Western herbs, chelation, hypnotherapy, biofeedback, supplements, dietary changes, group therapy and much, much more all have a place in a complementary medicine or a functional medicine approach.

Acceptance (mental state) - not defeat

I always say, 'make friends with reality'. Accepting that we don't live in the most brain-friendly environment is critical for gaining improvements. If you're in denial about your actual screen use, the effects are still happening, even while you deny it. It's pretty common. And it's important for us to accept our situation, day-by-day, minute-by-minute. Why? Because otherwise we are 'biting our own neck' (a wonderful expression!). You cannot start from where you are NOT. Start from where you are.

Body Work

From the Feldenkrais method (which has astonishing results for people with TBI) to massage to Rolfing, there are many modes of bodywork that can be useful in healing TBI. Just the physical touch of another can be an organizing force for the healing brain. At the very least, deep relaxation is a powerful tool.

Breathing Exercises

Breathing can be part of meditation techniques and used for relaxation. Actually, the possibilities are far greater than 'relaxation'. Wim Hof (known as the Iceman) has shown incredible physical capability, and increased mental fortitude through his breathing techniques and cold immersion. Probably we don't know exactly how certain breathwork can improve health and emotional states, but any type of deep breathing or yogic breathing seems to help.

Cervical Manual Therapy

This is a great therapy for those recovering from brain injury. The mechanics of most injuries means the cervical spine was involved. Another recommendation from the 2017 Berlin Consensus.

Cold Therapy

Great for your brain. Not a new therapy for TBI! The most basic understanding is that cold therapy reduces inflammation. We used ice packs around the neck and head for Aidan's recovery. There is a cryo helmet available online for more high-tech applications of cold. This consistently reduced symptoms, especially headache, disorientation and fatigue. Do not attempt cold water immersion without an assistant!

Diet

"Eat food. Not too much. Mostly plants." - Michael Pollan See the Primal Protocol for specifics.

Exercise

Research shows that exercise restores myelin, increases Brain-Derived Neurotrophic Factor (BDNF) and increases mitochondrial activity - all great things for brain health. Get some.

For those recovering from brain injury, the 2017 Berlin Consensus Statement recommends guided exercise as a concussion treatment that is supported by research. Controlled sub-symptom-threshold guided submaximal exercise is one of the most well researched beneficial treatments for concussion recovery.

Functional Medicine Approach

Functional medicine is medical practice or treatments that focus on optimal functioning of the body and its organs, usually involving systems of holistic or alternative medicine. There are multiple doctors, and providers that work through this paradigm. Some, like the Cerebrum Health Centers, have had great success with all types of patients.

Gratitude 'Exercises'

I am not going to cite research here. In any situation, gratitude can make it better. Read Viktor Frankl's book, *Man's Search for Meaning*.

Learn Something New

Should it surprise us that learning something new is good for the brain? Probably not. From building new neural networks to improving mood, engaging in learning has positive benefits for everyone.

Light Therapy

I insist that everyone read *The Brain's Way of Healing* by Dr. Norman Doidge. There are multiple studies on various wavelengths of light (cold lasers) in clinical settings and their application for TBI are just being rediscovered in the U.S. Biohackers are taking to the interwebs to showcase their use of red light (there are multiple types of red light devices for purchase) to improve sleep, immunity and more. To me, one of the most interesting facts is that light does penetrate the skull and plays an important role in brain health.

Meditation

Meditation, in its many forms, is helpful to the brain. It organizes brain waves and offers respite from our noisy world. You can use meditation apps like Headspace or learn from a teacher or learn on your own by reading or watching tutorials on YouTube.

Psychological/Cognitive Behavior Therapy

This is well-known and well-researched to help people recovering from brain injury. This is another recommendation from the 2017 Berlin Consensus Statement.

Rest

Rest is critical to the health and healing of the brain as well as all other physical systems. Just follow the brain's lead and rest as necessary. Why do I need to even say this? Because we live in a chronically sleep-deprived culture where about forty percent of the population gets less-than-recommended amounts of sleep.

Social Support

Whether you are the 'patient' or a caregiver, you will need help and doing this alone will only increase stress and reduce healing. Whether it's through church, work, a non-profit or extended family get help with meals, bills, childcare and anything else that needs attention. Social support includes joining support groups if those are available in your community. There are many online groups as well, some helpful, some not so much. Remember your mindset and don't expose yourself to negative people who don't believe in your healing.

Silence

Scientists found that mice who were 'exposed' to 2 hours of silence per day developed new cells in the hippocampus region of the brain (associated with memory, emotions and learning). Essentially, when we are not distracted by noise or tasks, quiet time allows the brain to process things. We may not think about it much, but our world is very noisy, just because we are accustomed to it doesn't mean our brain has 'adapted'.

UV Exposure (Sunlight)

Humans need light - real sunlight. Most post-TBI advice involves dark rooms and low 'stimulation'. However, human beings require UV light for total health, including important cell function. Dr. Jack Kruse is foremost in understanding how this process works. Real sunlight is necessary for healing, if not just for vitamin D levels but to also make sure melatonin production remains optimal.

Vestibular & Vision Therapy

Approximately thirty percent of patients will also have vestibular issues. Think dizziness/balance. However, zero percent of patients will require vestibular therapy alone, this must be paired with cervical and/or vision therapy to fully resolve. Also a recommendation from the 2017 Berlin Consensus.

Visualization Exercises

Whether it is to assist with a specific goal, or for overall healing, visualizing what you want helps get you there. There are different techniques, as well as guided visualization - take your pick. If you have trouble with driving spend five minutes a day visualizing driving well. If the issue is social situations, fantasize about having one great social interaction. In general, you can imagine the brain reducing inflammation or connecting neurons. This gives your brain a chance to practice the desired outcome.

CONCLUSION

Having a brain that is diminished or negatively impacted in any way is awful. Even brain fog is an impediment to our best selves. I really do believe that we can heal, we can improve and we can beat our man-made environment that is causing a lot of these negative downstream issues. From nutrition to neuroplasticity to exercise to light therapy - there is an answer that will improve not just brain health, but our entire wellbeing. It's not always easy, and it requires experimentation, but the brain is just an organ. If you can improve digestion or liver function, you can improve your brain. And you better. It's the only one you've got.

PRIMAL BRAIN REFERENCES

Ainsworth, C. (2015). Head Trauma Treatment and Management. Retrieved from http://emedicine.medscape.com/article/433855-treatment

Allred, R., Kim, S. & Jones, T. (2014). Use it and/or lose it—experience effects on brain remodeling across time after stroke. Frontiers in Human Neuroscience, 27 June 2014. https://doi.org/10.3389/fnhum.2014.00379

Berlin Consensus Statement. (2017). Consensus statement on concussion. Retrieved https://bjsm.bmj.com/content/early/2017/04/27/bjsports-2017-09769 9

Bernreuter, H. (2017). Head injuries to female athletes a troubling trend in MHSAA concussion study. MLive Media Group.

Bethune, B. (2015). How your brain heals itself. Retrieved from http://www.macleans.ca/society/health/how-your-brain-heals-itself/

Biello, D. (2016). Much of what we know about the brain may be wrong: The problem with fMRI. Retrieved from http://ideas.ted.com/much-of-what-we-know-about-the-brain-may-be-wrong-the-problem-with-fmri/

Blaylock, R. & Maroon, J. (2011). Immunoexcitotoxicity as a central mechanism in chronic traumatic encephalopathy-A unifying hypothesis. Surgical Neurology International. 2011;2:107. doi: 10.4103/2152-7806.83391.

Cardinale, A. (2016). Traumatic brain injury: The hidden epidemic nobody wants to talk about. Retrieved from http://psychcentral. com/blog/archives/2016/03/28/traumatic-brain-injury-the-hidden-epidemic-nobody-wants-to-talk-about/

Centers for Disease Control. (2014). TBI Data and Statistics. Retrieved from http://www.cdc.gov/TraumaticBrainInjury/data/index.html

Cha, A.E. (2017). There's Evidence That ADHD Could Be a Type of Sleep Disorder. Retrieved from http://www.sciencealert.com/there-s-evidence-that-adhd-could-be-a-type-of-sleep-disorder

Chih-Hung, K. et al. (2009). Brain activities associated with gaming Urge of online gaming addiction." Journal of Psychiatric Research. 43, 7:739–747. doi:10.1016/j.jpsychires.2008.09.012

Chuan-Bo, W., et al. (2013). Gray matter and white matter abnormalities in online game addiction." European Journal of Radiology 82, 8:1308–1312. doi:10.1016/j.ejrad.2013.01.031.

Doidge, N. (2016). The Brain's Way of Healing. Penguin Books, 2017.

Dunckley, V. (2014). Gray matters: Too much screen time damages the brain. Retrieved from https://www.psychologytoday.com/blog/mental-wealth/201402/gray-matters-too-much-screen-time-damages-the-brain

Elizabeth, E. (2017). 34 scientific studies showing adverse health effects from WIFI. Retrieved from https://www.healthnutnews.com/34-

scientific-studies-showing-adverse-health-effects-wi-fi/

Epstein, D. (2017). When Evidence Says No, But Doctors Say Yes. Retrieved from https://www.theatlantic.com/health/archive/2017/02/when-evidence-says-no-but-doctors-say-yes/517368/

Epstein, R. (2016). The Empty Brain. Retrieved from https://aeon.co/essays/your-brain-does-not-process-information-and-it-is-not-a-computer

French, L. (2015). Military Traumatic Brain Injury. Retrieved from http://www.brainlinemilitary.org/content/2011/01/military-traumatic-brain-injury-an-examination-of-important-differences_pageall.html

Fuchun, L. et al. (2012). Abnormal white matter integrity in adolescents with internet addiction disorder: A tract-based spatial statistics study." PloS One 7, 1:e30253. doi:10.1371/journal.pone.0030253.

Gornall, J. (2014). Will we ever understand the human brain? Retrieved from https://www.weforum.org/agenda/2014/09/understanding-human-brain/

Guangheng, D., Devito, E., Du, X., & Cui, Z. (2012) Impaired inhibitory control in 'Internet Addiction Disorder': A functional magnetic resonance imaging study." Psychiatry Research. 203, 2–3: 153–158. doi:10.1016/j.pscychresns.2012.02.001.

Guangheng, D., Hu, Y. & Lin, X. (2013). Reward/punishment sensitivities among internet addicts: Implications for their addictive behaviors." Progress in Neuro-Psychopharmacology & Biological Psychiatry. 46:139–145. doi:10.1016/j.pnpbp.2013.07.007

Haifeng, H., et al. (2012). Reduced striatal dopamine transporters in people with internet addiction disorder. Journal of Biomedicine & Biotechnology. doi:10.1155/2012/854524.

Hall, H. (2013). Dr. Amen's Love Affair with SPECT Scans. Retrieved from https://sciencebasedmedicine.org/dr-amens-love-affair-with-spect-scans/

Hamblin, J. (2014). The Toxins That Threaten Our Brains. Retrieved from https://www.theatlantic.com/health/archive/2014/03/the-toxins-that-threaten-our-brains/284466/

Han, D., et al. (2011). Brain activity and desire for internet video game play." Comprehensive Psychiatry. 52, 1:88–95. doi:10.1016/j.comppsych.2010.04.004.

Holland, M. (2017). Ketosis Aides in Protecting Against Traumatic Brain Injury. Retrieved from https://ketogenic.com/therapeutics/ketosis-aids-protecting-traumatic-brain-injury/

Kai, Y. (2013). et al. Cortical thickness abnormalities in late adolescence with online gaming addiction." Edited by Bogdan Draganski. PLoS ONE 8, 1. doi:10.1371/journal.pone.0053055.

Kühn, S., Romanowski, A. , Schilling, C. , Lorenz, R., et al. (2011). The neural basis of video gaming." Translational Psychiatry. 1:e53. doi:10.1038/tp.2011.53.

Logan, A. Katzman, M. & Balanza-Martinez, B. (2015). Natural environments, ancestral diets, and microbial ecology: Is there a modern "paleo-deficit disorder"? Part I. Journal of Physiological Anthropology.

2015; 34(1). doi: 10.1186/s40101-015-0041-y

Morley, W. & Seneff, S. (2014). Diminished brain resilience syndrome: A modern day neurological pathology of increased susceptibility to mild brain trauma, concussion, and downstream neurodegeneration. Surgical Neurology International. 5; 97.

Rao, V. & Vaishnavi, S. (2015). The Traumatized Brain - A Family Guide to Understanding Mood, Memory, and Behavior after Brain Injury. Johns Hopkins University Press, Baltimore, MD.

Rideout, V., Foehr, U. & Roberts, D. (2010). Generation M2: Media in the lives of 8- to 18- year olds. Kaiser Family Foundation Study. Retrieved from http://kff.org/other/poll-finding/report-generation-m2-media-in-the-lives/.

Sang Hee, K. (2011). Reduced striatal dopamine D2 receptors in people with internet addiction." Neuroreport. 22, 8:407–411. doi:10.1097/WNR.0b013e328346e16e.

Sciencealert. (2016). A bug in fMRI research could invalidate 15 years of brain research. Retrieved from http://www.sciencealert.com/a-bug-in-fmri-software-could-invalidate-decades-of-brain-research-scientists-discover

Science Daily. (2010). Vitamin D deficiency associated with chronic fatigue in brain injured patients. Retrieved from https://www.sciencedaily.com/releases/2010/04/100427182609.htm

Soon-Beom, H., et al. (2013). Decreased functional brain connectivity in adolescents with internet addiction. Edited by Xi-Nian Zuo. PLoS

ONE 8, 2. doi:10.1371/journal.pone.0057831.

Soon-Beom, H., et al. (2013). Reduced orbitofrontal cortical thickness in male adolescents with internet addiction." Behavioral and Brain Functions 9, 1. doi:10.1186/1744-9081-9-11.

Straus, L. 2015. When CT or MRI are Recommended After Concussion. Retrieved from http://www.momsteam.com/health-safety/ct-or-mri-usually-normal-after-concussion-but-recommended-in-some-circumstances

Sutherland, M. (2011). You're Grounded. Utne Reader. Retrieved from http://www.utne.com/mind-and-body/earthing-grounding-sleep-research-electromagnetic-fields

Traumatic Brain Injury. (2015). What is traumatic brain injury? Retrieved from http://www.traumaticbraininjury.com/understanding-tbi/what-is-traumatic-brain-injury/

Urban, T. (2017). Neuralink and the Brain's Magical Future. Retrieved from http://waitbutwhy.com/2017/04/neuralink.html

Virgin, JJ. (2017). Miracle Mindset. New York, North Star Way.

Williams, F. (2016). This is your brain on nature. Retrieved from http://www.nationalgeographic.com/magazine/2016/01/call-to-wild/

Yan, Z. et al. (2011). Gray matter abnormalities in internet addiction: A voxel-based morphometry study. European Journal of Radiology. 79, 1:92–95. doi:10.1016/j.ejrad.2009.10.025.

Zarkadakis, G. (2015). In Our Own Image. Pegasus Books, New York.

APPENDIX ONE

I recommend doing a side-by-side timeline to more objectively assess what is and what has been going on with your brain. It's a simple, but time-consuming, process. You have two columns, one is for events and one is for symptoms. Enter everything in chronological order. Under events, enter anything significant that you think has affected your health or life - this can be a chemical exposure, head injury, divorce, medical treatment, etc. Include the approximate date. Under symptoms, list symptoms as best you can, in order of their appearance in your life.

Sample:

EVENT	SYMPTOMS
1980 - Fell on pavement, hit back of head	Headache, dizziness, nausea and then sleep disturbances
1986 - Hit head on carnival ride	Headache, threw up, no further symptoms
1990 - General anesthesia	Recovery was slow, suffered uncommon depression afterwards

Made in the USA
San Bernardino, CA
05 January 2019